Physics, Pharmacology and Physiology for Anaesthetists

Key concepts for the FRCA

Physics, Pharmacology and Physiology for Anaesthetists

Key concepts for the FRCA

Matthew E. Cross MB ChB MRCP FRCA
Specialist Registrar in Anaesthetics, Queen Alexandra Hospital, Portsmouth, UK

Emma V. E. Plunkett MBBS MA MRCP FRCA
Specialist Registrar in Anaesthetics, St Mary's Hospital, London, UK

Foreword by

Tom E. Peck MBBS BSc FRCA
Consultant Anaesthetist, Royal Hampshire County Hospital, Winchester, UK

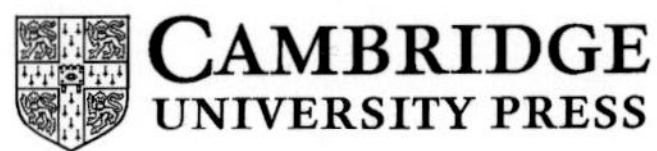

CAMBRIDGE UNIVERSITY PRESS
Cambridge, New York, Melbourne, Madrid, Cape Town, Singapore, São Paulo, Delhi

Cambridge University Press
The Edinburgh Building, Cambridge CB2 8RU, UK

Published in the United States of America by Cambridge University Press, New York

www.cambridge.org
For information on this title: www.cambridge.org/9780521700443

First published 2008
Reprinted 2009

Printed in the United Kingdom at the University Press, Cambridge

A catalogue record for this publication is available from the British Library

ISBN 978-0-521-70044-3 paperback

To Anna and Harvey for putting up with it all
and for Dad

MC

For all my family
but especially for Adrian

EP

Contents

Acknowledgements

We are grateful to the following individuals for their invaluable help in bringing this book to publication

Dr Tom Peck MBBS BSc FRCA
Anaesthetics Department, Royal Hampshire County Hospital, Winchester, UK

Dr David Smith DM FRCA
Shackleton Department of Anaesthetics, Southampton General Hospital, Southampton, UK

Dr Tom Pierce MRCP FRCA
Shackleton Department of Anaesthetics, Southampton General Hospital, Southampton, UK

Dr Mark du Boulay BSc FRCA
Anaesthetics Department, Royal Hampshire County Hospital, Winchester, UK

Dr Roger Sharpe BSc FRCA
Anaesthetics Department, Northwick Park Hospital, London, UK

In addition we are grateful for permission to reprint the illustrations on pages 183 and 184 from International Thomson Publishing Services Ltd.
Cheriton House, North Way, Andover, UK

Preface

The examinations in anaesthesia are much feared and respected. Although fair, they do require a grasp of many subjects which the candidate may not have been familiar with for some time. This is particularly true with regards to the basic science components.

This book does not aim to be an all-inclusive text, rather a companion to other books you will already have in your collection. It aims to allow you to have an additional reference point when revising some of these difficult topics. It will enable you to quickly and easily bring to hand the key illustrations, definitions or derivations that are fundamental to the understanding of a particular subject. In addition to succinct and accurate definitions of key phrases, important equations are derived step by step to aid understanding and there are more than 180 diagrams with explanations throughout the book.

You should certainly find a well-trusted textbook of anaesthesia if you wish to delve deeper into the subject matter, but we hope to be able to give you the knowledge and reasoning to tackle basic science MCQs and, more crucially, to buy you those first few lines of confident response when faced with a tricky basic science viva.

Good luck in the examinations, by the time you read this the end is already in sight!

Foreword

Many things are currently in a state of flux within the world of medical education and training, and the way in which candidates approach examinations is no exception. Gone are the days when large weighty works are the first port of call from which to start the learning experience. Trainees know that there are more efficient ways to get their heads around the concepts that are required in order to make sense of the facts.

It is said that a picture says a thousand words and this extends to diagrams as well. However, diagrams can be a double-edged sword for trainees unless they are accompanied by the relevant level of detail. Failure to label the axis, or to get the scale so wrong that the curve becomes contradictory is at best confusing.

This book will give back the edge to the examination candidate if they digest its contents. It is crammed full of precise, clear and well-labelled diagrams. In addition, the explanations are well structured and leave the reader with a clear understanding of the main point of the diagram and any additional information where required. It is also crammed full of definitions and derivations that are very accessible.

It has been pitched at those studying for the primary FRCA examination and I have no doubt that they will find it a useful resource. Due to its size, it is never going to have the last word, but it is not trying to achieve that. I am sure that it will also be a useful resource for those preparing for the final FRCA and also for those preparing teaching material for these groups.

Doctors Cross and Plunkett are to be congratulated on preparing such a clear and useful book – I shall be recommending it to others.

Dr Tom E. Peck MBBS BSc FRCA

Consultant Anaesthetist, Royal Hampshire County Hospital, Winchester, UK

Introduction

This book is aimed primarily at providing a reference point for the common graphs, definitions and equations that are part of the FRCA syllabus. In certain situations, for example the viva sections of the examinations, a clear structure to your answer will help you to appear more confident and ordered in your response. To enable you to do this, you should have a list of rules to hand which you can apply to any situation.

Graphs

Any graph should be constructed in a logical fashion. Often it is the best-known curves that candidates draw most poorly in their rush to put the relationship down on paper. The oxyhaemoglobin dissociation curve is a good example. In the rush to prove what they know about the subject as a whole, candidates often supply a poorly thought out sigmoid-type curve that passes through none of the traditional reference points when considered in more detail. Such an approach will not impress the examiner, despite a sound knowledge of the topic as a whole. Remembering the following order may help you to get off to a better start.

Size

It is important to draw a large diagram to avoid getting it cluttered. There will always be plenty of paper supplied so don't be afraid to use it all. It will make the examiner's job that much easier as well as yours.

Axes

Draw straight, perpendicular axes and label them with the name of the variable and its units before doing anything else. If common values are known for the particular variable then mark on a sensible range, for example 0–300 mmHg for blood pressure. Remember that logarithmic scales do not extend to zero as zero is an impossible result of a logarithmic function. In addition, if there are important reference points they should be marked both on the axis and where two variables intersect on the plot area, for example 75% saturation corresponding to 5.3 kPa for the venous point on the oxyhaemoglobin dissociation curve. Do all of this before considering a curve and do not be afraid to talk out loud as you do so – it avoids uncomfortable silences, focuses your thoughts and shows logic.

Beginning of a curve

Consider where a curve actually starts on the graph you are drawing. Does it begin at the origin or does it cross the y axis at some other point? If so, is there a specific value at which it crosses the y axis and why is that the case? Some curves do not come into contact with either axis, for example exponentials and some physiological autoregulation curves. If this is the case, then you should demonstrate this fact and be ready to explain why it is so. Consider what happens to the slope of a curve at its extremes. It is not uncommon for a curve to flatten out at high or low values, and you should indicate this if it is the case.

Middle section

The middle section of a curve may cross some important points as previously marked on the graph. Make sure that the curve does, in fact, cross these points rather than just come close to them or you lose the purpose of marking them on in the first place. Always try to think what the relationship between the two variables is. Is it a straight line, an exponential or otherwise and is your curve representing this accurately?

End of a curve

If the end of a curve crosses one of the axes then draw this on as accurately as possible. If it does not reach an axis then say so and consider what the curve will look like at this extreme.

Other points

Avoid the temptation to overly annotate your graphs but do mark on any important points or regions, for example segments representing zero and first-order kinetics on the Michaelis–Menten graph.

Definitions

When giving a definition, the aim is to *accurately* describe the principle in question in as few a words as possible. The neatness with which your definition appears will affect how well considered your answer as a whole comes across. Definitions may or may not include units.

Definitions containing units

Always think about what units, if any, are associated with the item you are trying to describe. For example, you know that the units for clearance are $ml.min^{-1}$ and so your definition must include a statement about both volume (ml) and time (min). When you are clear about what you are describing, it should be presented as succinctly as possible in a format such as

'*x*' is the **volume** of plasma ...
'*y*' is the **pressure** found when ...
'*z*' is the **time** taken for ...
Clearance **(ml.min^{-1})** is the volume **(ml)** of plasma from which a drug is completely removed per unit time **(min)**
Pressure **(N.m^{-2})** describes the result of a force **(N)** being applied over a given area **(m^2)**.

You can always finish your definition by offering the units to the examiner if you are sure of them.

Definitions without units

If there are no units involved, think about what process you are being asked to define. It may be a ratio, an effect, a phenomenon, etc.

Reynold's number is a **dimensionless number** ...
The blood:gas partition coefficient is the **ratio** of ...
The second gas effect is the **phenomenon** by which ...

Conditions

Think about any conditions that must apply. Are the measurements taken at standard temperature and pressure (STP) or at the prevailing temperature and pressure?

The triple point of water is the temperature at which all three phases are in equilibrium at **611.73 Pa. It occurs at 0.01 °C.**

There is no need to mention a condition if it does not affect the calculation. For example, there is no need to mention ambient pressure when defining saturated vapour pressure (SVP) as only temperature will alter the SVP of a volatile.

Those definitions with clearly associated units will need to be given in a clear and specific way; those without units can often be 'padded' a little if you are not entirely sure.

Equations

Most equations need only be learned well enough to understand the components which make up the formula such as in

$$V = IR$$

where V is voltage, I is current and R is resistance.

There are, however, some equations that deserve a greater understanding of their derivation. These include,

The Bohr equation
The Shunt equation
The Henderson–Hasselbach equation

These equations are fully derived in this book with step by step explanations of the mathematics involved. It is unlikely that the result of your examination will hinge on whether or not you can successfully derive these equations from first principles, but a knowledge of how to do it will make things clearer in your own mind.

If you are asked to derive an equation, remember four things.

1. Don't panic!
2. Write the end equation down **first** so that the examiners know you know it.
3. State the first principles, for example the Bohr equation considers a single tidal exhalation comprising both dead space and alveolar gas.
4. Attempt to derive the equation.

If you find yourself going blank or taking a wrong turn midway through then do not be afraid to tell the examiners that you cannot remember and would they mind moving on. No one will mark you down for this as you have already supplied them with the equation and the viva will move on in a different direction.

Mathematical relationships

Mathematical relationships tend not to be tested as stand-alone topics but an understanding of them will enable you to answer other topics with more authority.

Linear relationships

$y = x$

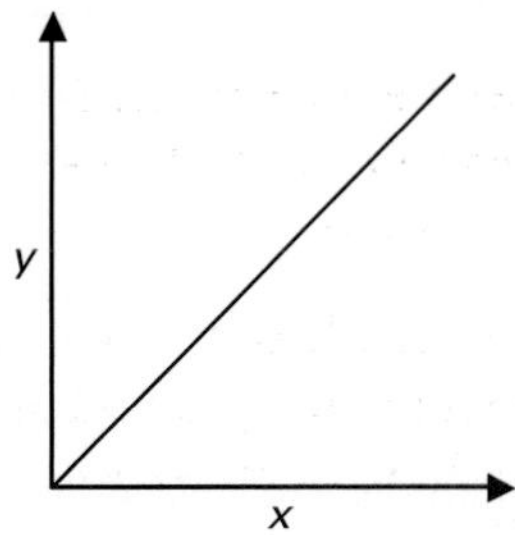

Draw and label the axes as shown. Plot the line so that it passes through the origin (the point at which both x and y are zero) and the value of y is equal to the value of x at every point. The slope when drawn correctly should be at 45° if the scales on both axes are the same.

$y = ax + b$

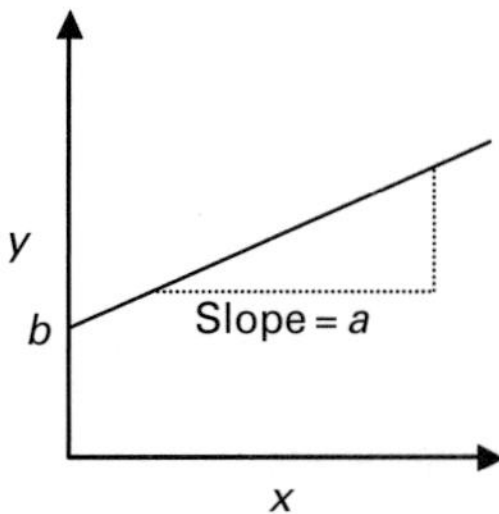

This line should cross the y axis at a value of b because when x is 0, y must be $0 + \mathrm{b}$. The slope of the graph is given by the multiplier a. For example, when the equation states that $y = 2x$, then y will be 4 when x is 2, and 8 when x is 4, etc. The slope of the line will, therefore, be twice as steep as that of the line given by $y = 1x$.

Hyperbolic relationships ($y=k/x$)

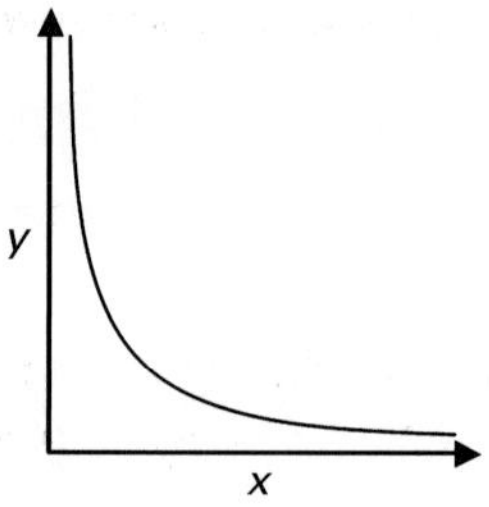

This curve describes any inverse relationship. The commonest value for the constant, k, in anaesthetics is 1, which gives rise to a curve known as a rectangular hyperbola. The line never crosses the x or the y axis and is described as asymptotic to them (see definition below). Boyle's law is a good example (volume = 1/pressure). This curve looks very similar to an exponential decline but they are entirely different in mathematical terms so be sure about which one you are describing.

Asymptote

A curve that continually approaches a given line but does not meet it at any distance.

Parabolic relationships ($y=kx^2$)

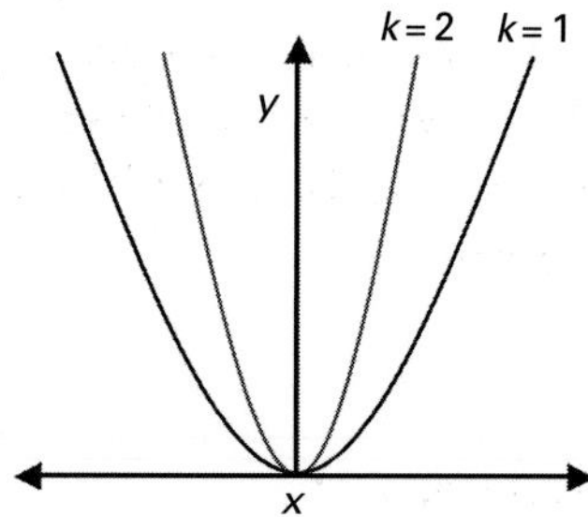

These curves describe the relationship $y=x^2$ and so there can be no negative value for y. The value for 'k' alters the slope of the curve, as 'a' does for the equation $y=ax+b$. The curve crosses the y axis at zero unless the equation is written $y=kx^2+b$, in which case it crosses at the value of 'b'.

Exponential relationships and logarithms

Exponential

A condition where the rate of change of a variable at any point in time is proportional to the value of the variable at that time.

or

A function whereby the x variable becomes the exponent of the equation $y = e^x$.

We are normally used to x being represented in equations as the *base* unit (i.e. $y = x^2$). In the exponential function, it becomes the exponent ($y = e^x$), which conveys some very particular properties.

Euler's number

Represents the numerical value 2.71828 and is the base of natural logarithms. Represented by the symbol 'e'.

Logarithms

The power (x) to which a base must be raised in order to produce the number given as for the equation $x = \log_{\text{base}}(\text{number})$.

The base can be any number, common numbers are 10, 2 and e (2.71828). $\text{Log}_{10}(100)$ is, therefore, the power to which 10 must be raised to produce the number 100; for $10^2 = 100$, therefore, the answer is $x = 2$. Log_{10} is usually written as log whereas $\log_e$ is usually written ln.

Rules of logarithms

Multiplication becomes addition

$$\log(xy) = \log(x) + \log(y)$$

Division becomes subtraction

$$\log(x/y) = \log(x) - \log(y)$$

Reciprocal becomes negative

$$\log(1/x) = -\log(x)$$

Power becomes multiplication

$$\log(x^n) = n.\log(x)$$

Any log of its own base is one

$$\log_{10}(10) = 1 \text{ and } \ln(e) = 1$$

Any log of 1 is zero because n^0 always equals 1

$$\log_{10}(1) = 0 \text{ and } \ln(1) = 0$$

Basic positive exponential ($y = e^x$)

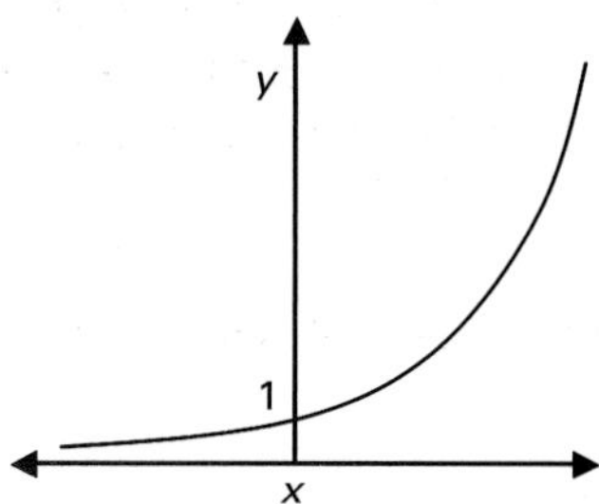

The curve is asymptotic to the x axis. At negative values of x, the slope is shallow but the gradient increases sharply when x is positive. The curve intercepts the y axis at 1 because any number to the power 0 (as in e^0) equals 1. Most importantly, the value of y at any point equals the slope of the graph at that point.

Clinical tear away positive exponential ($y = a.e^{kt}$)

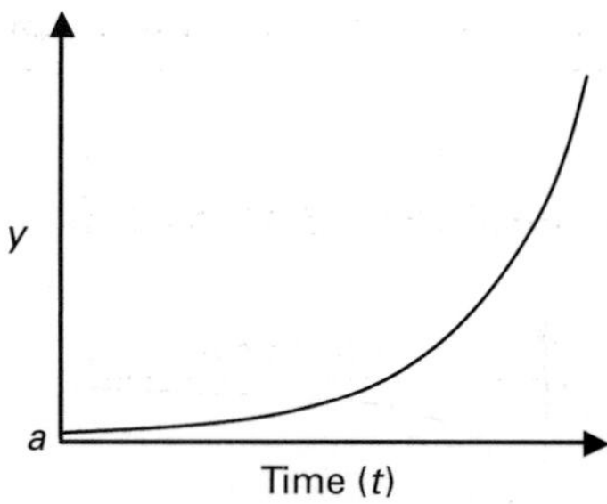

The curve crosses y axis at value of a. It tends towards infinity as value of t increases. This is clearly not a sustainable physiological process but could be seen in the early stages of bacterial replication where y equals number of bacteria.

Basic negative exponential ($y=a^{-x}$)

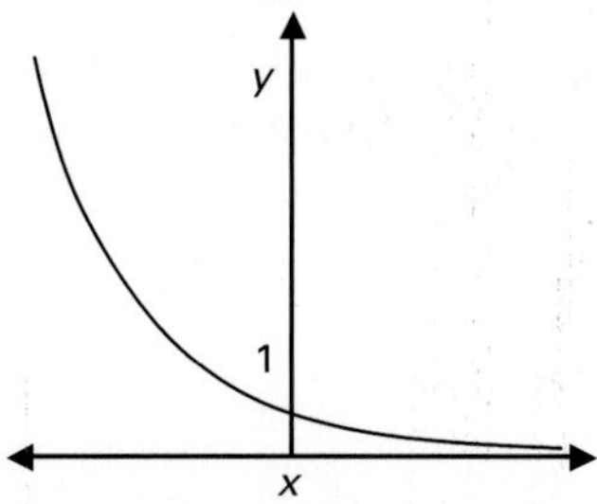

The x axis is again an asymptote and the line crosses the y axis at 1. This time the curve climbs to infinity as x becomes more negative. This is because $-x$ is now becoming more positive. The curve is simply a mirror image, around the y axis, of the positive exponential curve seen above.

Physiological negative exponential ($y=a.\mathrm{e}^{-kt}$)

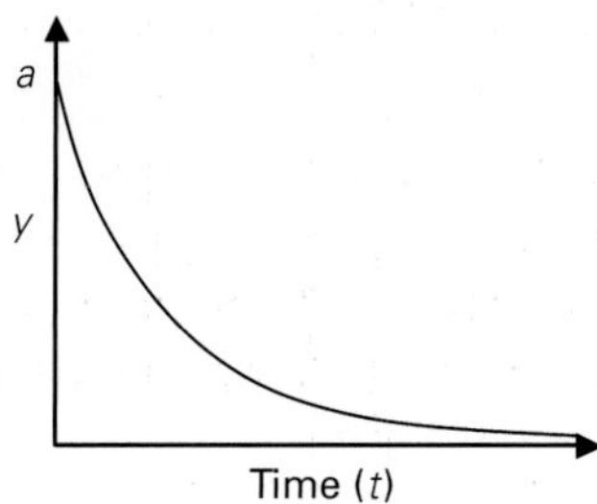

The curve crosses the y axis at a value of a. It declines exponentially as t increases. The line is asymptotic to the x axis. This curve is seen in physiological processes such as drug elimination and lung volume during passive expiration.

Physiological build-up negative exponential ($y=a-b.\mathrm{e}^{-kt}$)

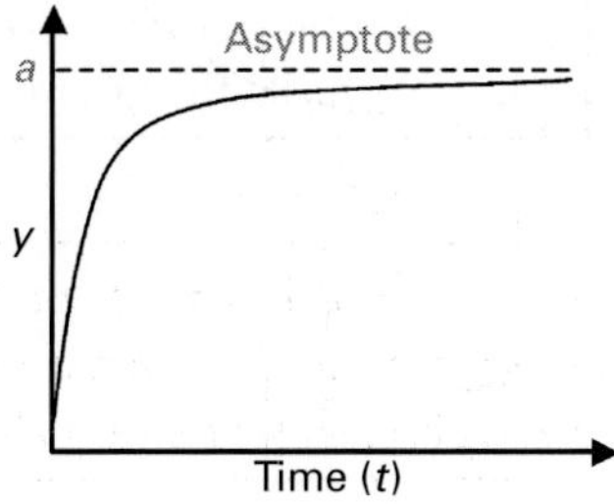

The curve passes through the origin and has an asymptote that crosses the y axis at a value of a. Although y increases with time, the curve is actually a negative exponential. This is because the *rate* of increase in y is decreasing exponentially as t increases. This curve may be seen clinically as a wash-in curve or that of lung volume during positive pressure ventilation using pressure-controlled ventilation.

Half life

> The time taken for the value of an exponential function to decrease by half is the half life and is represented by the symbol $t_{1/2}$
>
> or
>
> the time equivalent of 0.693τ $\quad\quad$ τ=*time constant*

An exponential process is said to be complete after five half lives. At this point, 96.875% of the process has occurred.

Graphical representation of half life

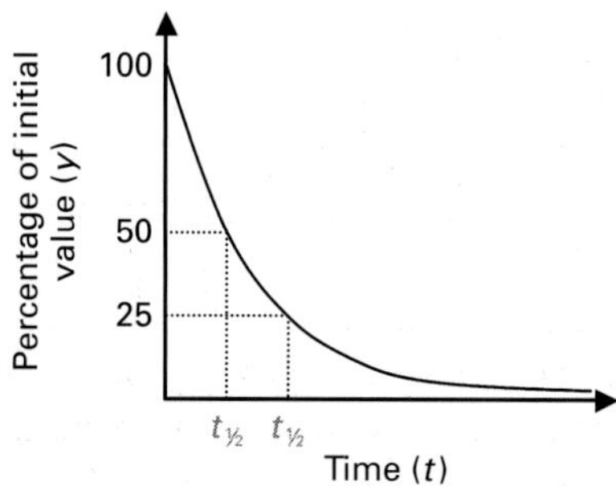

This curve needs to be drawn accurately in order to demonstrate the principle. After drawing and labelling the axes, mark the key values on the y axis as shown. Your curve must pass through each value at an equal time interval on the x axis. To ensure this, plot equal time periods on the x axis as shown, before drawing the curve. Join the points with a smooth curve that is asymptotic to the x axis. This will enable you to describe the nature of an exponential decline accurately as well as to demonstrate easily the meaning of half life.

Time constant

> The time it would have taken for a negative exponential process to complete, were the initial rate of change to be maintained throughout. Given the symbol τ.
>
> or
>
> The time taken for the value of an exponential to fall to 37% of its previous value.
>
> or
>
> The time taken for the value of an exponential function change by a factor of e^1.
>
> or
>
> The reciprocal of the rate constant.

An exponential process is said to be complete after three time constants. At this point 94.9% of the process has occurred.

Graphical representation of the time constant

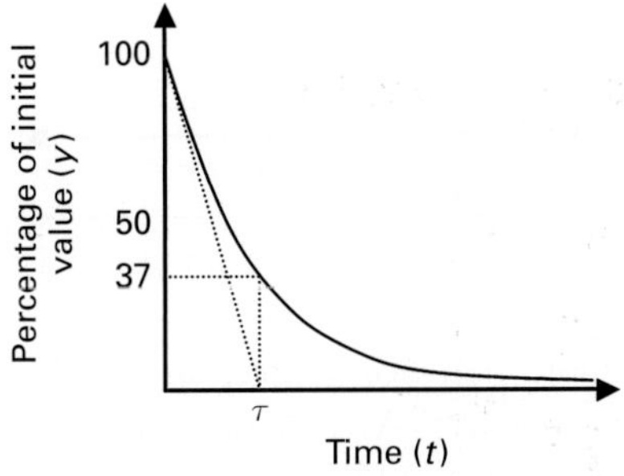

This curve should be a graphical representation of the first and second definitions of the time constant as given above. After drawing and labelling the axes, mark the key points on the y axis as shown. Draw a straight line falling from 100 to baseline at a time interval of your choosing. Label this time interval τ. Mark a point on the graph where a vertical line from this point crosses 37% on the y axis. Finally draw the curve starting as a tangent to your original straight line and falling away smoothly as shown. Make sure it passes through the 37% point accurately. A well-drawn curve will demonstrate the time constant principle clearly.

Rate constant

> The reciprocal of the time constant. Given the symbol k.
> or
> A marker of the rate of change of an exponential process.

The rate constant acts as a modifier to the exponent as in the equation $y = e^{kt}$ (e.g. in a savings account, k would be the interest rate; as k increases, more money is earned in the same period of time and the exponential curve is steeper).

Graphical representation of k ($y = e^{kt}$)

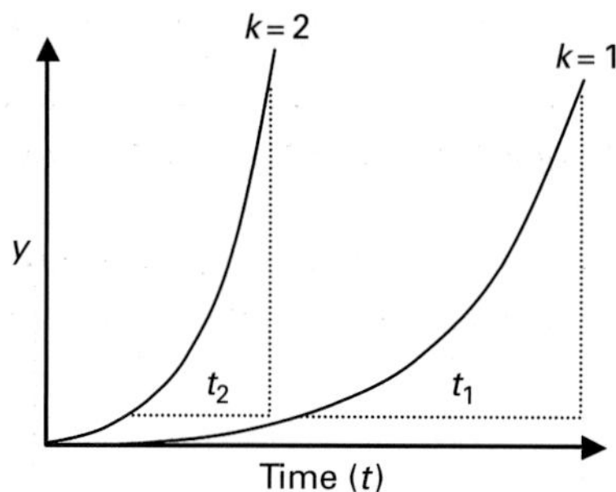

$k = 1$ Draw a standard exponential tear-away curve. To move from $y = e^t$ to $y = e^{t+1}$ takes time t_1. **$k = 2$** This curve should be twice as steep as the first as 'k' acts as a 2× multiplier to the exponent 't'. As 'k' has doubled, for the same change in y the time taken has halved and this can be shown as t_2 where t_2 is half the value of t_1. The values t_1 and t_2 are also the time constants for the equation because they are, by definition, the reciprocal of the rate constant.

Transforming to a straight line graph

Start with the general equation as follows

$$y = e^{kt}$$

take natural logarithms of both sides

$$\ln y = \ln(e^{kt})$$

power functions become multipliers when taking logs, giving

$$\ln y = kt.\ln(e)$$

the natural log of e is 1, giving

$$\ln y = kt.1 \text{ or } \ln y = kt$$

You may be expected to perform this simple transformation, or at least to describe the maths behind it, as it demonstrates how logarithmic transformation can make the interpretation of exponential curves much easier by allowing them to be plotted as straight lines $\ln y = kt$.

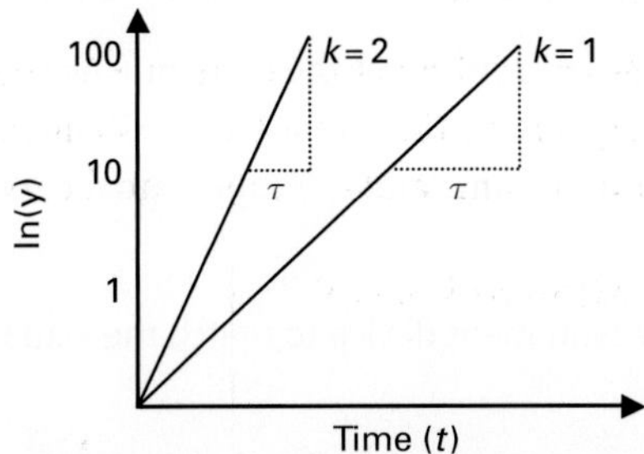

$k = 1$ Draw a curve passing through the origin and rising as a straight line at approximately 45°.
$k = 2$ Draw a curve passing through the origin and rising twice as steeply as the $k = 1$ line. The time constant is half that for the $k = 1$ line.

Physical measurement and calibration

This topic tests your understanding of the ways in which a measurement device may not accurately reflect the actual physiological situation.

Accuracy

The ability of a measurement device to match the actual value of the quantity being measured.

Precision

The reproducibility of repeated measurements and a measure of their likely spread.

In the analogy of firing arrows at a target, the accuracy would represent how close the arrow was to the bullseye, whereas the precision would be a measure of how tightly packed together a cluster of arrows were once they had all been fired.

Drift

A fixed deviation from the true value at all points in the measured range.

Hysteresis

The phenomenon by which a measurement varies from the input value by different degrees depending on whether the input variable is increasing or decreasing in magnitude at that moment in time.

Non-linearity

The absence of a true linear relationship between the input value and the measured value.

Zeroing and calibration

Zeroing a display removes any fixed drift and allows the accuracy of the measuring system to be improved. If all points are offset by '$+x$', zeroing simply subtracts 'x' from all the display values to bring them back to the input value. Calibration is used to check for linearity over a given range by taking known set points and checking that they all display a measured value that lies on the ideal straight line. The more points that fit the line, the more certain one can be that the line is indeed straight. One point calibration reveals nothing about linearity, two point calibration is better but the line may not necessarily be straight outside your two calibration points (even a circle will cross the straight line at two points). Three point calibration is ideal as, if all three points are on a straight line, the likelihood that the relationship is linear over the whole range is high.

Accurate and precise measurement

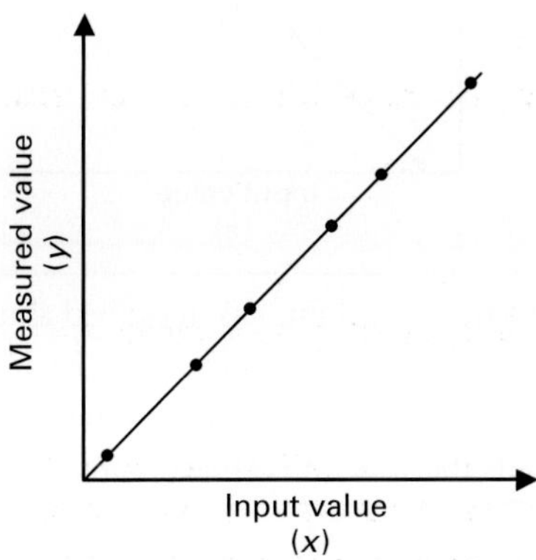

Draw a straight line passing through the origin so that every input value is exactly matched by the measured value. In mathematical terms it is the same as the curve for $y = x$.

Accurate imprecise measurement

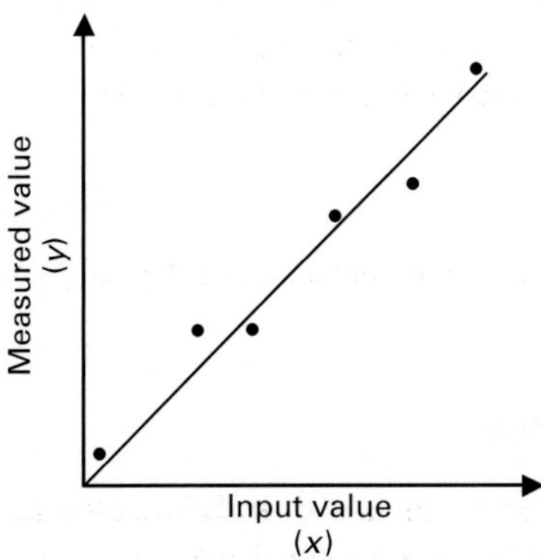

Draw the line of perfect fit as described above. Each point on the graph is plotted so that it lies away from this line (imprecision) but so that the line of best fit matches the perfect line (accuracy).

Precise inaccurate measurement

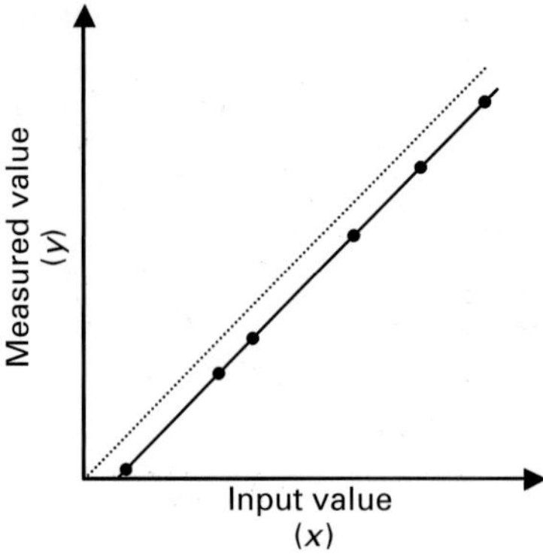

Draw the line of perfect fit (dotted line) as described above. Next plot a series of measured values that lie on a parallel (solid) line. Each point lies exactly on a line and so is precise. However, the separation of the measured value from the actual input value means that the line is inaccurate.

Drift

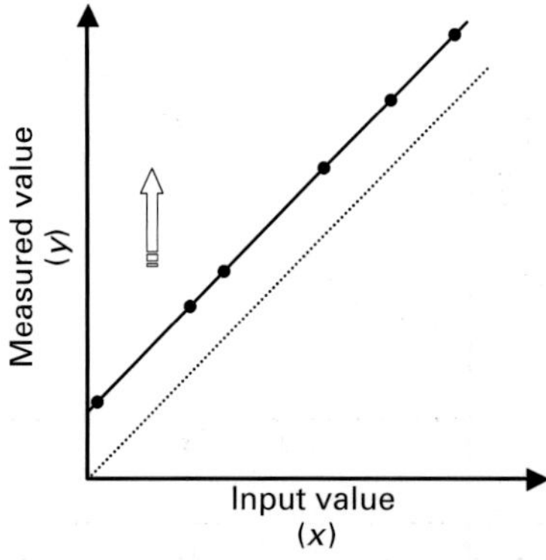

The technique is the same as for drawing the graph above. Demonstrate that the readings can be made accurate by the process of zeroing – altering each measured value by a set amount in order to bring the line back to its ideal position. The term 'drift' implies that accuracy is lost over time whereas an inaccurate implies that the error is fixed.

Hysteresis

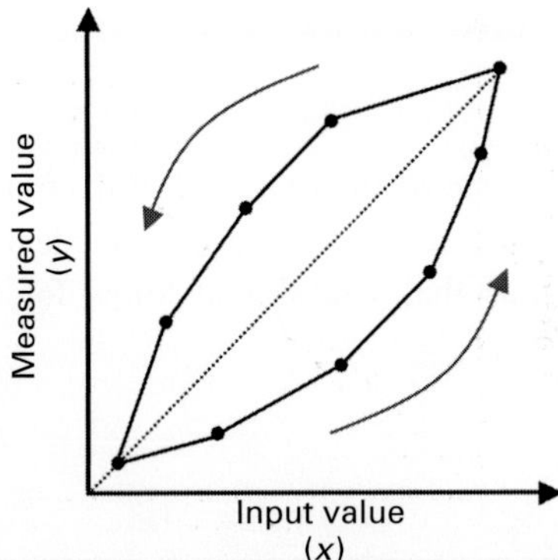

The curves should show that the measured value will be different depending on whether the input value is increasing (bottom curve) or decreasing (top curve). Often seen clinically with lung pressure–volume curves.

Non-linearity

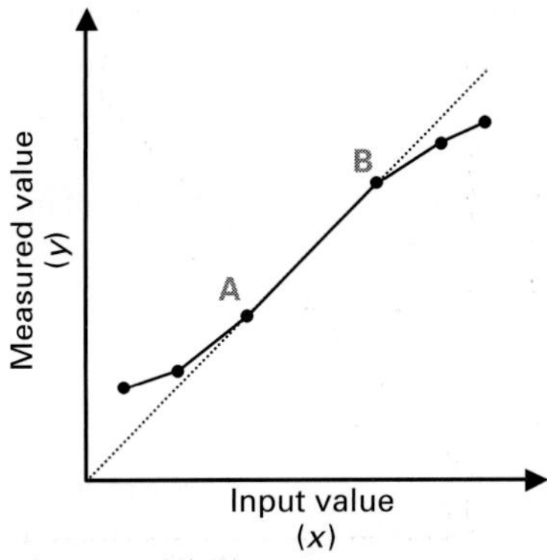

The curve can be any non-linear shape to demonstrate the effect. The curve helps to explain the importance and limitations of calibration. Points A and B represent a calibration range of input values between which linearity is likely. The curve demonstrates how linearity cannot be assured outside this range. The DINAMAP monitor behaves in a similar way. It tends to overestimate at low blood pressure (BP) and underestimate at high BP while retaining accuracy between the calibration limits.

The SI units

There are seven basic SI (Système International) units from which all other units can be derived. These seven are assumed to be independent of each other and have various specific definitions that you should know for the examination. The acronym is SMMACKK.

The base SI units

Unit	Symbol	Measure of	Definition
second	s	Time	The duration of a given number of oscillations of the caesium-133 atom
metre	m	Distance	The length of the path travelled by light in vacuum during a certain fraction of a second
mole	mol	Amount	The amount of substance which contains as many elementary particles as there are atoms in 0.012 kg of carbon-12
ampere	A	Current	The current in two parallel conductors of infinite length and placed 1 metre apart in vacuum, which would produce between them a force of 2×10^{-7} N.m^{-1}
candela	cd	Luminous intensity	Luminous intensity, in a given direction, of a source that emits monochromatic light at a specific frequency
kilogram	kg	Mass	The mass of the international prototype of the kilogram held in Sèvres, France
kelvin	K	Temperature	1/273.16 of the thermodynamic temperature of the triple point of water

From these seven base SI units, many others are derived. For example, speed can be denoted as distance per unit time (m.s^{-1}) and acceleration as speed change per unit time (m.s^{-2}). Some common derived units are given below.

Derived SI units

Measure of	Definition	Units
Area	Square metre	m^2
Volume	Cubic metre	m^3
Speed	Metre per second	$m.s^{-1}$
Velocity	Metre per second in a given direction	$m.s^{-1}$
Acceleration	Metre per second squared	$m.s^{-2}$
Wave number	Reciprocal metre	m^{-1}
Current density	Ampere per square metre	$A.m^2$
Concentration	Mole per cubic metre	$mol.m^{-3}$

These derived units may have special symbols of their own to simplify them. For instance, it is easier to use the symbol Ω than $m^2.kg.s^{-3}.A^{-2}$.

Derived SI units with special symbols

Measure of	Name	Symbol	Units
Frequency	hertz	Hz	s^{-1}
Force	newton	N	$kg.m.s^{-2}$
Pressure	pascal	Pa	$N.m^{-2}$
Energy/work	joule	J	N.m
Power	watt	W	$J.s^{-1}$
Electrical charge	coulomb	C	A.s
Potential difference	volt	V	W/A
Capacitance	farad	F	C/V
Resistance	ohm	Ω	V/A

Some everyday units are recognized by the system although they themselves are not true SI units. Examples include the litre (10^{-3} m^3), the minute (60 s), and the bar (10^5 Pa). One litre is the volume occupied by 1 kg of water but was redefined in the 1960s as being equal to 1000 cm^3.

Prefixes to the SI units

In reality, many of the SI units are of the wrong order of magnitude to be useful. For example, a pascal is a tiny amount of force (imagine 1 newton – about 100 g – acting on an area of 1 m^2 and you get the idea). We, therefore, often use kilopascals (kPa) to make the numbers more manageable. The word kilo- is one of a series of prefixes that are used to denote a change in the order of magnitude of a unit. The following prefixes are used to produce multiples or submultiples of all SI units.

Prefixes

Prefix	10^n	Symbol	Decimal equivalent
yotta	10^{24}	Y	1 000 000 000 000 000 000 000 000
zetta	10^{21}	Z	1 000 000 000 000 000 000 000
exa	10^{18}	E	1 000 000 000 000 000 000
peta	10^{15}	P	1 000 000 000 000 000
tera	10^{12}	T	1 000 000 000 000
giga	10^{9}	G	1 000 000 000
mega	10^{6}	M	1 000 000
kilo	10^{3}	k	1000
hecto	10^{2}	h	100
deca	10^{1}	da	10
	10^{0}		1
deci	10^{-1}	d	0.1
centi	10^{-2}	c	0.01
milli	10^{-3}	m	0.001
micro	10^{-6}	μ	0.000 001
nano	10^{-9}	n	0.000 000 001
pico	10^{-12}	p	0.000 000 000 001
femto	10^{-15}	f	0.000 000 000 000 001
atto	10^{-18}	a	0.000 000 000 000 000 001
zepto	10^{-21}	z	0.000 000 000 000 000 000 001
yocto	10^{-24}	y	0.000 000 000 000 000 000 000 001

Interestingly, 10^{100} is known as a googol, which was the basis for the name of the internet search engine Google after a misspelling occurred.

Simple mechanics

Although there is much more to mechanics as a topic, an understanding of some of its simple components (force, pressure, work and power) is all that will be tested in the examination.

Force

Force is that influence which tends to change the state of motion of an object (newtons, N).
or

$$F = ma$$

where F is force, m is mass and a is acceleration.

Newton

That force which will give a mass of one kilogram an acceleration of one metre per second per second
or

$$N = kg.m.s^{-2}$$

When we talk about weight, we are really discussing the force that we sense when holding a mass which is subject to acceleration by gravity. The earth's gravitational field will accelerate an object at 9.81 $m.s^{-2}$ and is, therefore, equal to 9.81 N. If we hold a 1 kg mass in our hands we sense a 1 kg weight, which is actually 9.81 N:

$$F = ma$$
$$F = 1\,kg \times 9.81\,m.s^{-2}$$
$$F = 9.81\,N$$

Therefore, 1 N is 9.81 times less force than this, which is equal to a mass of 102 g (1000/9.81). Putting it another way, a mass of 1 kg will not weigh 1 kg on the moon as the acceleration owing to gravity is only one-sixth of that on the earth. The 1 kg mass will weigh only 163 g.

Pressure

Pressure is force applied over a unit area (pascals, P)

$$P = F/A$$

P is pressure, F is force and A is area.

Pascal

One pascal is equal to a force of one newton applied over an area of one square metre ($N.m^{-2}$).

The pascal is a tiny amount when you realize that 1 N is equal to 102 g weight. For this reason kilopascals (kPa) are used as standard.

Energy

The capacity to do work (joules, J).

Work

Work is the result of a force acting upon an object to cause its displacement in the direction of the force applied (joules, J).
or

$$J = FD$$

J is work, F is force and D is distance travelled in the direction of the force.

Joule

The work done when a force of one newton moves one metre in the direction of the force is one joule.

More physiologically, it can be shown that work is given by pressure × volume. This enables indices such as work of breathing to be calculated simply by studying the pressure–volume curve.

$$P = F/A \quad \text{or} \quad F = PA$$

and

$$V = DA \quad \text{or} \quad D = V/A$$

so

$$J = FD$$

becomes

$$J = (PA).(V/A)$$

or

$$J = PV$$

where P is pressure, F is force, A is area, V is volume, D is distance and J is work.

Power

The rate at which work is done (watts, W).
or

$$\mathrm{W} = \mathrm{J/s}$$

where W is watts (power), J is joules (work) and s is seconds (time).

Watt

The power expended when one joule of energy is consumed in one second is one watt.

The power required to sustain physiological processes can be calculated by using the above equation. If a pressure–volume loop for a respiratory cycle is plotted, the work of breathing may be found. If the respiratory rate is now measured then the power may be calculated. The power required for respiration is only approximately 700–1000 mW, compared with approximately 80 W needed at basal metabolic rate.

The gas laws

Boyle's law

At a constant temperature, the volume of a fixed amount of a perfect gas varies inversely with its pressure.

$$PV = K \text{ or } V \propto 1/P$$

Charles' law

At a constant pressure, the volume of a fixed amount of a perfect gas varies in proportion to its absolute temperature.

$$V/T = K \text{ or } \mathrm{V} \propto \mathrm{T}$$

Gay–Lussac's law (The third gas law)

At a constant volume, the pressure of a fixed amount of a perfect gas varies in proportion to its absolute temperature.

$$P/T = K \text{ or } P \propto T$$

Remember that water *Boyle's* at a constant temperature and that Prince *Charles* is under constant pressure to be king.

Perfect gas

A gas that completely obeys all three gas laws.
or
A gas that contains molecules of infinitely small size, which, therefore, occupy no volume themselves, and which have no force of attraction between them.

It is important to realize that this is a theoretical concept and no such gas actually exists. Hydrogen comes the closest to being a perfect gas as it has the lowest molecular weight. In practice, most commonly used anaesthetic gases obey the gas laws reasonably well.

Avogadro's hypothesis

Equal volumes of gases at the same temperature and pressure contain equal numbers of molecules.

The universal gas equation

The universal gas equation combines the three gas laws within a single equation

If $PV = K_1$, $P/T = K_2$ and $V/T = K_3$, then all can be combined to give

$$PV/T = K$$

For 1 mole of a gas, K is named the universal gas constant and given the symbol R.

$$PV/T = R$$

for n moles of gas

$$PV/T = nR$$

so

$$PV = nRT$$

The equation may be used in anaesthetics when calculating the contents of an oxygen cylinder. The cylinder is at a constant (room) temperature and has a fixed internal volume. As R is a constant in itself, the only variables now become P and n so that

$$\mathrm{P} \propto \mathrm{n}$$

Therefore, the pressure gauge can be used as a measure of the amount of oxygen left in the cylinder. The reason we cannot use a nitrous oxide cylinder pressure gauge in the same way is that these cylinders contain both vapour and liquid and so the gas laws do not apply.

Laminar flow

Laminar flow describes the situation when any fluid (either gas or liquid) passes smoothly and steadily along a given path, this is is described by the Hagen–Poiseuille equation.

Hagen–Poiseuille equation

$$Flow = \frac{\pi p r^4}{8\eta l}$$

where p is pressure drop along the tube $(p_1 - p_2)$, r is radius of tube, l is length of tube and η is viscosity of fluid.

The most important aspect of the equation is that flow is proportional to the 4th power of the radius. If the radius doubles, the flow through the tube will increase by 16 times (2^4).

Note that some texts describe the equation as

$$\text{Flow} = \frac{\pi p d^4}{128\eta l}$$

where d is the diameter of tube.

This form uses the diameter rather than the radius of the tube. As the diameter is twice the radius, the value of d^4 is 16 times (2^4) that of r^4. Therefore, the constant (8) on the bottom of the equation must also be multiplied 16 times to ensure the equation remains balanced ($8 \times 16 = 128$).

Viewed from the side as it is passing through a tube, the leading edge of a column of fluid undergoing laminar flow appears parabolic. The fluid flowing in the centre of this column moves at twice the average speed of the fluid column as a whole. The fluid flowing near the edge of the tube approaches zero velocity. This phenomenon is particular to laminar flow and gives rise to this particular shape of flow.

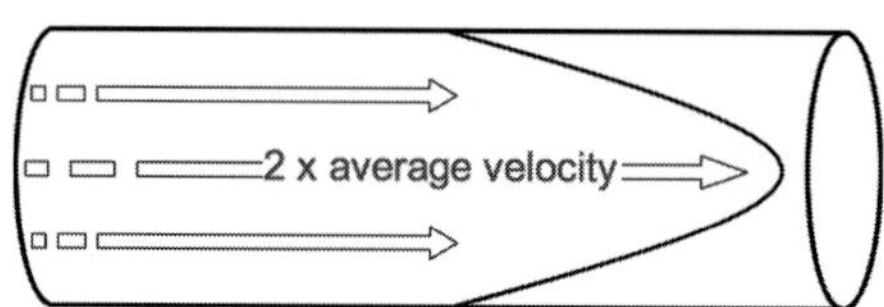

Turbulent flow

Turbulent flow describes the situation in which fluid flows unpredictably with multiple eddy currents and is not parallel to the sides of the tube through which it is flowing.

As flow is, by definition, unpredictable, there is no single equation that defines the rate of turbulent flow as there is with laminar flow. However, there is a number that can be calculated in order to identify whether fluid flow is likely to be laminar or turbulent and this is called Reynold's number (*Re*).

Reynold's number

$$Re = \frac{\rho v d}{\eta}$$

where Re is Reynold's number, ρ is density of fluid, v is velocity of fluid, d is diameter of tube and η is viscosity of fluid.

If one were to calculate the units of all the variables in this equation, you would find that they all cancel each other out. As such, Reynold's number is dimensionless (it has no units) and it is simply taken that

when $Re < 2000$ flow is *likely* to be laminar and when $Re > 2000$ flow is *likely* to be turbulent.

Given what we now know about laminar and turbulent flow, the main points to remember are that

viscosity is the important property for laminar flow
density is the important property for turbulent flow
Reynold's number of 2000 delineates laminar from turbulent flow.

Bernoulli, Venturi and Coanda

The Bernoulli principle

An increase in the flow velocity of an ideal fluid will be accompanied by a simultaneous reduction in its pressure.

The Venturi effect

The effect by which the introduction of a constriction to fluid flow within a tube causes the velocity of the fluid to increase and, therefore, the pressure of the fluid to fall.

These definitions are both based on the law of conservation of energy (also known as the 'first law of thermodynamics').

The law of conservation of energy

Energy cannot be created or destroyed but can only change from one form to another.

Put simply, this means that the total energy contained within the fluid system must always be constant. Therefore, as the kinetic energy (velocity) of the fluid increases, the potential energy (pressure) must reduce by an equal amount in order to ensure that the total energy content remains the same.

The increase in velocity seen as part of the Venturi effect simply demonstrates that a given number of fluid particles have to move faster through a narrower section of tube in order to keep the total flow the same. This means an increase in velocity and, as predicted, a reduction in pressure. The resultant drop in pressure can be used to entrain gases or liquids, which allows for applications such as nebulizers and Venturi masks.

The Coanda effect

The tendency of a stream of fluid flowing in proximity to a convex surface to follow the line of the surface rather than its original course.

The effect is thought to occur because a moving column of fluid entrains molecules lying close to the curved surface, creating a relatively low pressure, contact point. As the pressure further away from the curved surface is relatively higher, the column of fluid is preferentially 'pushed' towards the surface rather than continuing its straight course. The effect means that fluid will preferentially flow down one limb of a Y-junction rather than being equally distributed.

Heat and temperature

Heat

The form of energy that passes between two samples owing to the difference in their temperatures.

Temperature

The property of matter which determines whether heat energy will flow to or from another object of a different temperature.

Heat energy will flow from an object of a high temperature to an object of a lower temperature. An object with a high temperature does not necessarily contain more heat energy than one with a lower temperature as the temperature change per unit of heat energy supplied will depend upon the specific heat capacity of the object in question.

Triple point

The temperature at which all three phases of water – solid, liquid and gas – are in equilibrium at 611.73 Pa. It occurs at 0.01 °C.

Kelvin

One kelvin is equal to 1/273.16 of the thermodynamic triple point of water. A change in temperature of 1 K is equal in magnitude to that of 1 °C.

Kelvin must be used when performing calculations with temperature. For example, the volume of gas at 20 °C is not double that at 10 °C: 10 °C is 283.15 K so the temperature must rise to 566.30 K (293.15 °C) before the volume of gas will double.

Celsius/centigrade

Celsius (formerly called the degree centigrade) is a common measure of temperature in which a change of 1 °C is equal in magnitude to a change of 1 K. To convert absolute temperatures given in degrees celsius to kelvin, you must add 273.15. For example 20 °C = 293.15 K.

Resistance wire

The underlying principle of this method of measuring temperature is that the resistance of a thin piece of metal increases as the temperature increases. This makes an extremely sensitive thermometer yet it is fragile and has a slow response time.

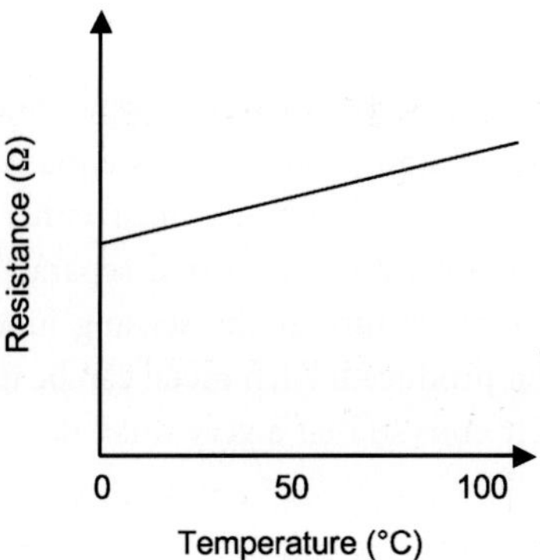

Draw a curve that does not pass through the origin. Over commonly measured ranges, the relationship is essentially linear. The slope of the graph is very slightly positive and a Wheatstone bridge needs to be used to increase sensitivity.

Thermistor

A thermistor can be made cheaply and relies on the fact that the resistance of certain semiconductor metals falls as temperature increases. Thermistors are fast responding but suffer from calibration error and deteriorate over time.

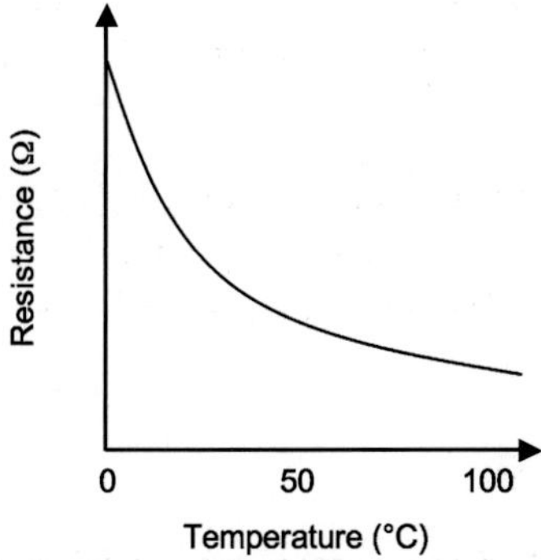

Draw a smooth curve that falls as temperature increases. The curve will never cross the x axis. Although non-linear, this can be overcome by mathematical manipulation.

The Seebeck effect

At the junction of two dissimilar metals, a voltage will be produced, the magnitude of which will be in proportion to the temperature difference between two such junctions.

Thermocouple

The thermocouple utilizes the Seebeck effect. Copper and constantan are the two metals most commonly used and produce an essentially linear curve of voltage against temperature. One of the junctions must either be kept at a constant temperature or have its temperature measured separately (by using a sensitive thermistor) so that the temperature at the sensing junction can be calculated according to the potential produced. Each metal can be made into fine wires that come into contact at their ends so that a very small device can be made.

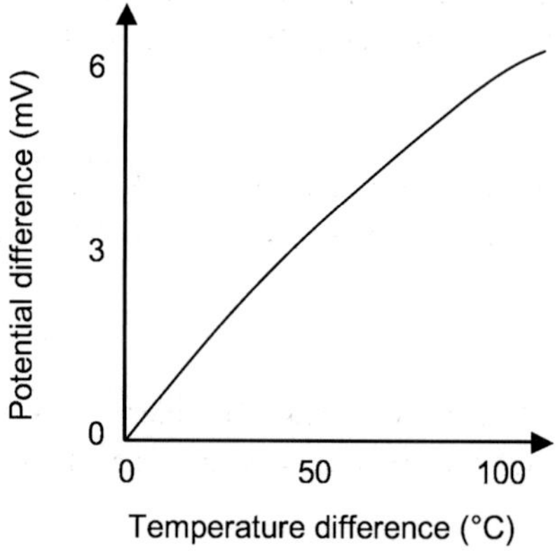

This curve passes through the origin because if there is no temperature difference between the junctions there is no potential generated. It rises as a near linear curve over the range of commonly measured values. The output voltage is small ($0.04–0.06\,mV.^{\circ}C^{-1}$) and so signal amplification is often needed.

Humidity

The term humidity refers to the amount of water vapour present in the atmosphere and is subdivided into two types:

Absolute humidity

The total mass of water vapour present in the air per unit volume ($kg.m^{-3}$ or $g.m^{-3}$).

Relative humidity

The ratio of the amount of water vapour in the air compared with the amount that would be present at the same temperature if the air was fully saturated. (RH, %)

or

The ratio of the vapour pressure of water in the air compared with the saturated vapour pressure of water at that temperature (%).

Dew point

The temperature at which the relative humidity of the air exceeds 100% and water condenses out of the vapour phase to form liquid (dew).

Hygrometer

An instrument used for measuring the humidity of a gas.

Hygroscopic material

One that attracts moisture from the atmosphere.

The main location of hygroscopic mediums is inside heat and moisture exchange (HME) filters.

Humidity graph

The humidity graph is attempting to demonstrate how a fixed amount of water vapour in the atmosphere will lead to a variable relative humidity depending on the prevailing temperature. It also highlights the importance of the upper airways in a room fully humidifying by the addition of 27 g.m^{-3} of water vapour. You will be expected to know the absolute humidity of air at body temperature.

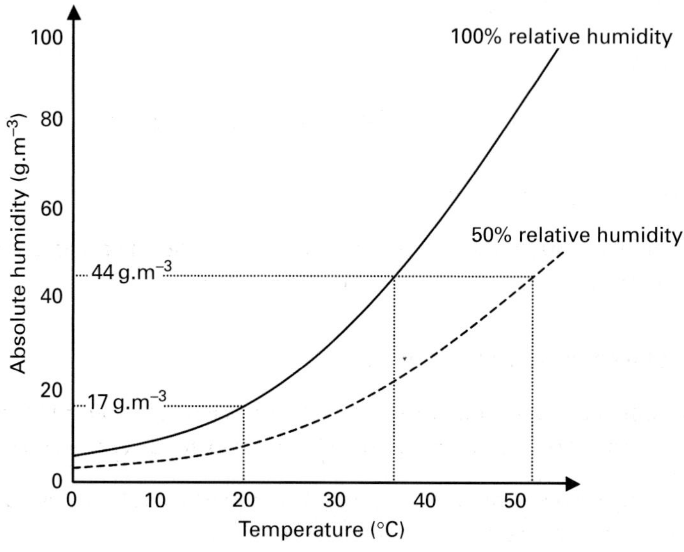

100% RH After drawing and labelling the axes, plot the key y values as shown. The 100% line crosses the y axis at 8 g.m^{-3} and rises as a parabola crossing the points shown. These points must be accurate.

50% RH This curve crosses each point on the x axis at a y value half that of the 100% RH line. Air at 50% RH cannot contain 44 g.m^{-3} water until over 50 °C. The graph demonstrates that a fixed quantity of water vapour can result in varying RH depending on the temperature concerned.

Latent heat

Not all heat energy results in a temperature change. In order for a material to change phase (solid, liquid, gas) some energy must be supplied to it to enable its component atoms to alter their arrangement. This is the concept of latent heat.

Latent heat

The heat energy that is required for a material to undergo a change of phase (J).

Specific latent heat of fusion

The amount of heat required, at a specified temperature, to convert a unit mass of solid to liquid without temperature change ($J.kg^{-1}$).

Specific latent heat of vaporization

The amount of heat energy required, at a specified temperature, to convert a unit mass of liquid into the vapour without temperature change ($J.kg^{-1}$).

Note that these same amounts of energy will be released into the surroundings when the change of phase is in the reverse direction.

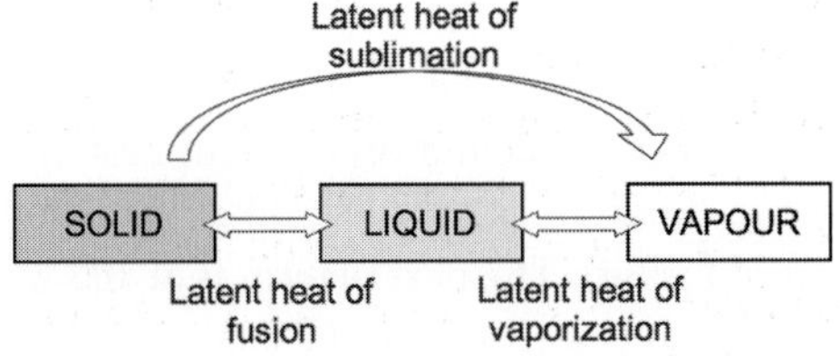

Heat capacity

The heat energy required to raise the temperature of a given object by one degree ($J.K^{-1}$ or $J.^{\circ}C^{-1}$).

Specific heat capacity

The heat energy required to raise the temperature of one kilogram of a substance by one degree ($J.kg^{-1}.K^{-1}$ or $J.kg^{-1}.^{\circ}C^{-1}$).

Specific heat capacity is a different concept to latent heat as it relates to an actual temperature change.

There is an important graph associated with the concept of latent heat. It is described as a heating curve and shows the temperature of a substance in relation to time. A constant amount of heat is being supplied per unit time and the main objective is to demonstrate the plateaus where phase change is occurring. At these points, the substance does not change its temperature despite continuing to absorb heat energy from the surroundings.

Heating curve for water

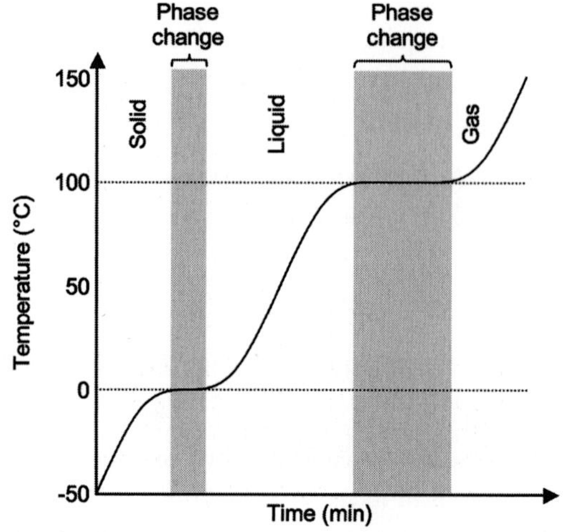

The curve crosses the *y* axis at a negative value of your choosing. Between the plateaus, the slope is approximately linear. The plateaus are crucial as they are the visual representation of the definition of latent heat. The first plateau is at 0 °C and is short in duration as only 334 $kJ.kg^{-1}$ is absorbed in this time (specific latent heat of fusion). The next plateau is at 100 °C and is longer in duration as 2260 $kJ.kg^{-1}$ is absorbed (specific latent heat of vaporization).

Isotherms

An isotherm is a line of constant temperature and it forms part of a diagram that shows the relationship between temperature, pressure and volume. The graph is gas specific and usually relates to nitrous oxide. Three lines are chosen to illustrate the volume–pressure relationship above, at and below the critical temperature.

Nitrous oxide isotherm

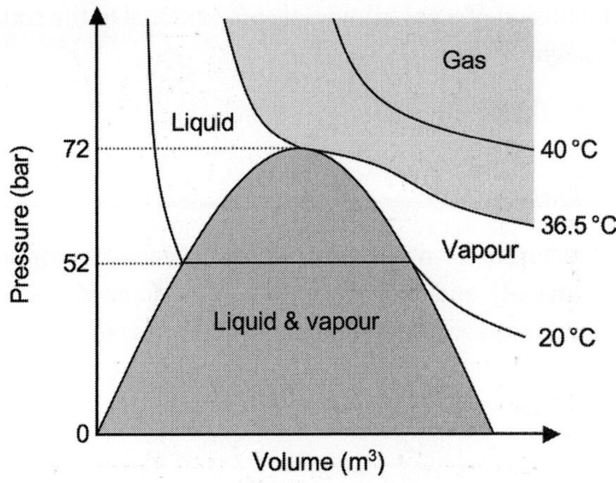

Liquid and vapour Draw this outline on the diagram first in order that your other lines will pass through it at the correct points.

20 °C From right to left, the line curves up initially and then becomes horizontal as it crosses the 'liquid/vapour' curve. Once all vapour has been liquidized, the line climbs almost vertically as liquid is incompressible, leading to a rapid increase in pressure for a small decrease in volume.

36.5 °C The critical temperature line. This climbs from right to left as a rectangular hyperbola with a small flattened section at its midpoint. This is where a small amount of gas is liquidized. It climbs rapidly after this section as before.

40 °C A true rectangular hyperbola representing Boyle's law. The pressure doubles as the volume halves. As it is above the critical temperature, it is a gas and obeys the gas laws.

Solubility and diffusion

Henry's law

The amount of gas dissolved in a liquid is directly proportional to the partial pressure of the gas in equilibrium with the liquid.

Graham's law

The rate of diffusion of a gas is inversely proportional to the square root of its molecular weight.

$$\text{Rate} \propto 1/\sqrt{\text{MW}}$$

Fick's law of diffusion

The rate of diffusion of a gas across a membrane is proportional to the membrane area (A) and the concentration gradient ($C_1 - C_2$) across the membrane and inversely proportional to its thickness (D).

$$\text{Rate of diffusion} \propto \frac{A[C_1 - C_2]}{D}$$

Blood : gas solubility coefficient

The ratio of the amount of substance present in equal volume phases of blood and gas in a closed system at equilibrium and at standard temperature and pressure.

Oil : gas solubility coefficient

The ratio of the amount of substance present in equal volume phases of oil and gas in a closed system at equilibrium and at standard temperature and pressure.

Bunsen solubility coefficient

The volume of gas, corrected to standard temperature and pressure, that dissolves in one unit volume of liquid at the temperature concerned where the partial pressure of the gas above the liquid is one atmosphere.

Ostwald solubility coefficient

> **The volume of gas that dissolves in one unit volume of liquid at the temperature concerned.**

The Ostwald solubility coefficient is, therefore, independent of the partial pressure.

Osmosis and colligative properties

Osmole

One osmole is an amount of particles equal to Avogadro's number (6.02×10^{23}).

Osmolarity

The amount of osmotically active particles present per litre of solution ($mmol.l^{-1}$).

Osmolality

The amount of osmotically active particles present per kilogram of solvent ($mmol.kg^{-1}$).

Osmotic pressure

The pressure exerted within a sealed system of solution in response to the presence of osmotically active particles on one side of a semipermeable membrane (kPa).

One osmole of solute exerts a pressure of 101.325 kPa when dissolved in 22.4 L of solvent at 0 °C.

Colligative properties

Those properties of a solution which vary according to the osmolarity of the solution. These are:

- depression of freezing point. The freezing point of a solution is depressed by 1.86 °C per osmole of solute per kilogram of solvent
- reduction of vapour pressure
- elevation of boiling point
- increase in osmotic pressure.

Raoult's law

The depression of freezing point or reduction of the vapour pressure of a solvent is proportional to the molar concentration of the solute.

Osmometer

An osmometer is a device used for measuring the osmolality of a solution. Solution is placed in the apparatus, which cools it rapidly to 0 °C and then supercools it more slowly to −7 °C. This cooling is achieved by the Peltier effect (absorption of heat at the junction of two dissimilar metals as a voltage is applied), which is the reverse of the Seebeck effect. The solution remains a liquid until a mechanical stimulus is applied, which initiates freezing. This is a peculiar property of the supercooling process. The latent heat of fusion is released during the phase change from liquid to solid so warming the solution until its natural freezing point is attained.

Graph

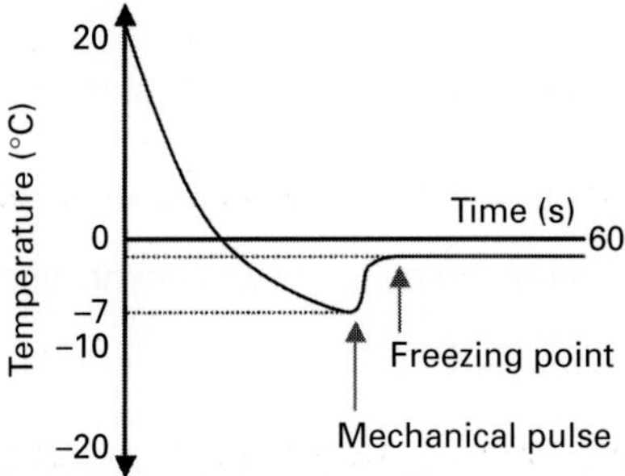

> Plot a smooth curve falling rapidly from room temperature to 0 °C. After this the curve flattens out until the temperature reaches −7 °C. Cooling is then stopped and a mechanical stirrer induces a pulse. The curve rises quickly to achieve a plateau temperature (freezing point).

Resistors and resistance

Electrical resistance is a broad term given to the opposition of flow of current within an electrical circuit. However, when considering components such as capacitors or inductors, or when speaking about resistance to alternating current (AC) flow, certain other terminology is used.

Resistance

The opposition to flow of direct current (ohms, Ω).

Reactance

The opposition to flow of alternating current (ohms, Ω).

Impedance

The total of the resistive and reactive components of opposition to electrical flow (ohms, Ω).

All three of these terms have units of ohms as they are all measures of some form of resistance to electrical flow. The reactance of an inductor is high and comes specifically from the back electromotive force (EMF; p. 46) that is generated within the coil. It is, therefore, difficult for AC to pass. The reactance of a capacitor is relatively low but its resistance can be high; therefore, direct current (DC) does not pass easily. Reactance does not usually exist by itself as each component in a circuit will generate some resistance to electrical flow. The choice of terms to define total resistance in a circuit is, therefore, resistance or impedance.

Ohm's law

The strength of an electric current varies directly with the electromotive force (voltage) and inversely with the resistance.

$$I = V/R$$

or

$$V = IR$$

where V is voltage, I is current and R is resistance.

The equation can be used to calculate any of the above values when the other two are known. When R is calculated, it may represent resistance or impedance depending on the type of circuit being used (AC/DC).

Capacitors and capacitance

Capacitor

A device that stores electrical charge.

A capacitor consists of two conducting plates separated by a non-conducting material called the dielectric.

Capacitance

The ability of a capacitor to store electrical charge (farads, F).

Farad

A capacitor with a capacitance of one farad will store one coulomb of charge when one volt is applied to it.

$$F = C/V$$

where F is farad (capacitance), C is coulomb (charge) and V is volt (potential difference).

One farad is a large value and most capacitors will measure in micro- or picofarads

Principle of capacitors

Electrical current is the flow of electrons. When electrons flow onto a plate of a capacitor it becomes negatively charged and this charge tends to drive electrons off the adjacent plate through repulsive forces. When the first plate becomes full of electrons, no further flow of current can occur and so current flow in the circuit ceases. The rate of decay of current is exponential. Current can only continue to flow if the polarity is reversed so that electrons are now attracted to the positive plate and flow off the negative plate.

The important point is that capacitors will, therefore, allow the flow of AC in preference to DC. Because there is less time for current to decay in a high-frequency AC circuit before the polarity reverses, the mean current flow is greater. The acronym **CLiFF** may help to remind you that **c**apacitors act as **l**ow-**f**requency **f**ilters in that they tend to oppose the flow of low frequency or DC.

Graphs show how capacitors alter current flow within a circuit. The points to demonstrate are that DC decays rapidly to zero and that the mean current flow is less in a low-frequency AC circuit than in a high-frequency one.

Capacitor in DC circuit

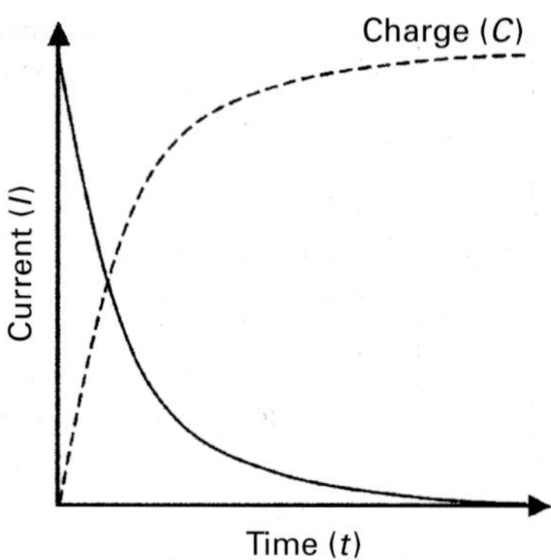

These curves would occur when current and charge were measured in a circuit containing a capacitor at the moment when the switch was closed to allow the flow of DC. Current undergoes an exponential decline, demonstrating that the majority of current flow occurs through a capacitor when the current is rapidly changing. The reverse is true of charge that undergoes exponential build up.

Capacitor in low-frequency AC circuit

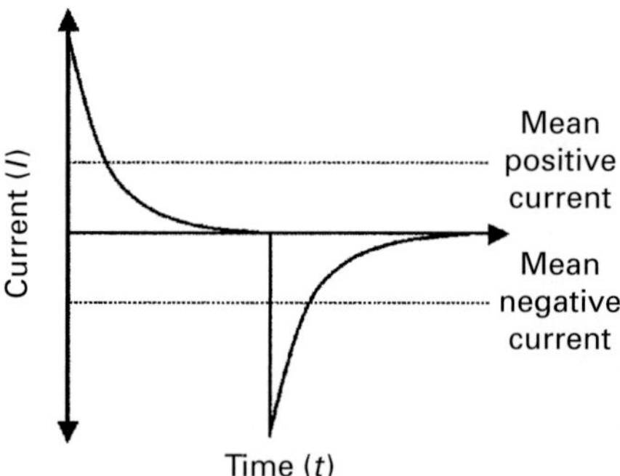

Base this curve on the previous diagram and imagine a slowly cycling AC waveform in the circuit. When current flow is positive, the capacitor acts as it did in the DC circuit. When the current flow reverses polarity the capacitor generates a curve that is inverted in relation to the first. The mean current flow is low as current dies away exponentially when passing through the capacitor.

Capacitor in high-frequency AC circuit

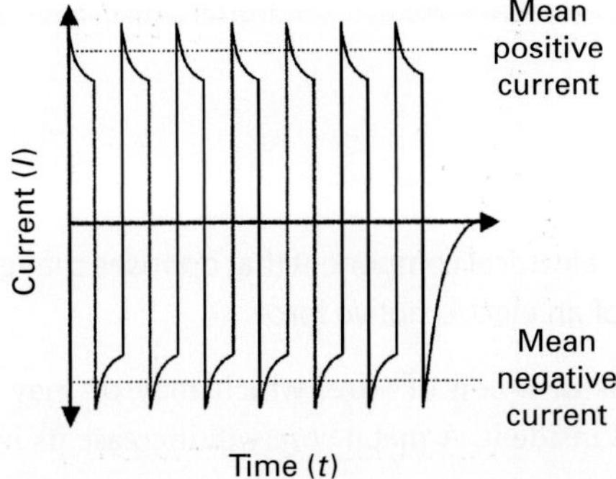

When the current in a circuit is alternating rapidly, there is less time for exponential decay to occur before the polarity changes. This diagram should demonstrate that the mean positive and negative current flows are greater in a high-frequency AC circuit.

Inductors and inductance

Inductor

An inductor is an electrical component that opposes changes in current flow by the generation of an electromotive force.

An inductor consists of a coil of wire, which may or may not have a core of ferromagnetic metal inside it. A metal core will increase its inductance.

Inductance

Inductance is the measure of the ability to generate a resistive electromotive force under the influence of changing current (henry, H).

Henry

One henry is the inductance when one ampere flowing in the coil generates a magnetic field strength of one weber.

$$H = Wb/A$$

where H is henry (inductance), Wb is weber (magnetic field strength) and A is ampere (current).

Electromotive force (EMF)

An analogous term to voltage when considering electrical circuits and components (volts, E).

Principle of inductors

A current flowing through any conductor will generate a magnetic field around the conductor. If any conductor is moved through a magnetic field, a current will be generated within it. As current flow through an inductor coil changes, it generates a changing magnetic field around the coil. This changing magnetic field, in turn, induces a force that acts to oppose the original current flow. This opposing force is known as the back EMF.

In contrast to a capacitor, an inductor will allow the passage of DC and low-frequency AC much more freely than high-frequency AC. This is because the amount of back EMF generated is proportional to the rate of change of the current through the inductor. It, therefore, acts as a high-frequency filter in that it tends to oppose the flow of high-frequency current through it.

Graphs

A graph of current flow versus time aims to show how an inductor affects current flow in a circuit. It is difficult to draw a graph for an AC circuit, so a DC example is often used. The key point is to demonstrate that the back EMF is always greatest when there is greatest change in current flow and so the amount of current successfully passing through the inductor at these points in time is minimal.

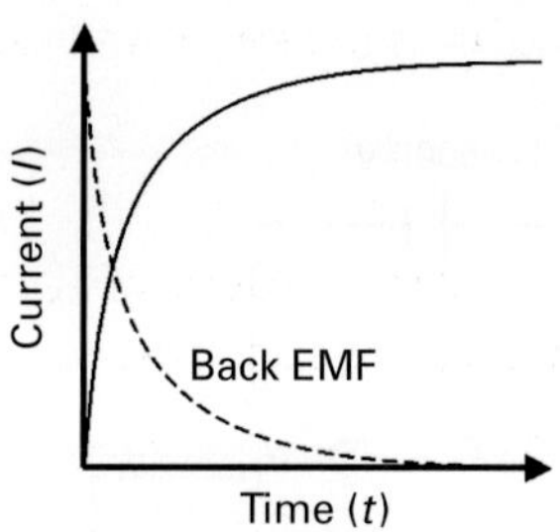

Current Draw a build-up exponential curve (solid line) to show how current flows when an inductor is connected to a DC source. On connection, the rate of change of current is great and so a high back EMF is produced. What would have been an instantaneous 'jump' in current is blunted by this effect. As the back EMF dies down, a steady state current flow is reached.

Back EMF Draw an exponential decay curve (dotted) to show how back EMF is highest when rate of change of current flow is highest. This explains how inductors are used to filter out rapidly alternating current in clinical use.

Defibrillators

Defibrillator circuit

You may be asked to draw a defibrillator circuit diagram in the examination in order to demonstrate the principles of capacitors and inductors.

Charging

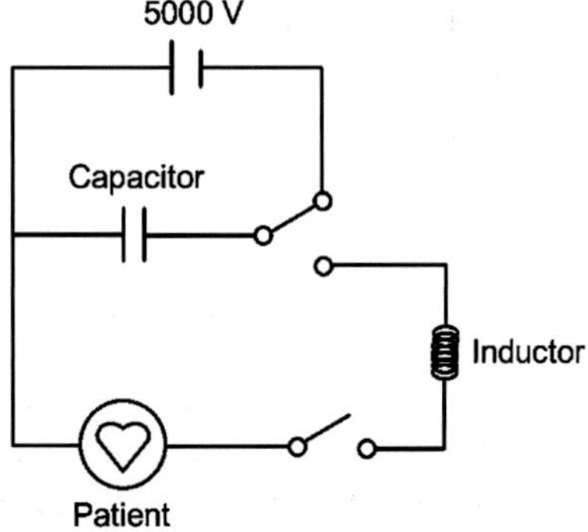

When charging the defibrillator, the switch is positioned so that the 5000 V DC current flows only around the upper half of the circuit. It, therefore, causes a charge to build up on the capacitor plates.

Discharging

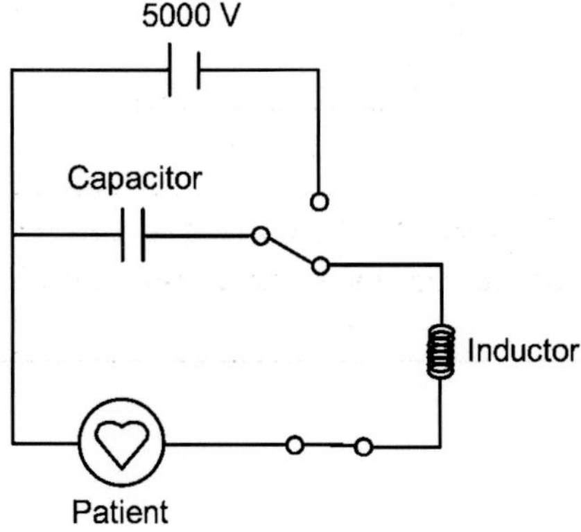

When discharging, the upper and lower switches are both closed so that the stored charge from the capacitor is now delivered to the patient. The inductor acts to modify the current waveform delivered as described below.

Defibrillator discharge

The inductor is used in a defibrillation circuit to modify the discharge waveform of the device so as to prolong the effective delivery of current to the myocardium.

Unmodified waveform

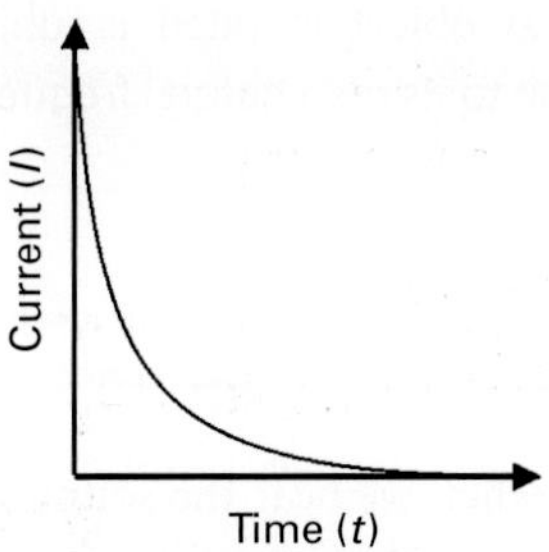

The unmodified curve shows exponential decay of current over time. This is the waveform that would result if there were no inductors in the circuit.

Modified waveform

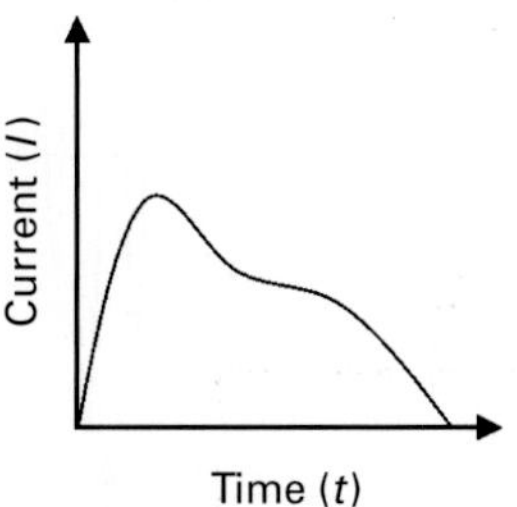

The modified waveform should show that the waveform is prolonged in duration after passing through the inductor and that it adopts a smoother profile.

Resonance and damping

Both resonance and damping can cause some confusion and the explanations of the underlying physics can become muddled in a viva situation. Although the deeper mathematics of the topic are complex, a basic understanding of the underlying principles is all the examiners will want to see.

Resonance

> The condition in which an object or system is subjected to an oscillating force having a frequency close to its own natural frequency.

Natural frequency

> The frequency of oscillation that an object or system will adopt freely when set in motion or supplied with energy (hertz, Hz).

We have all felt resonance when we hear the sound of a lorry's engine begin to make the window pane vibrate. The natural frequency of the window is having energy supplied to it by the sound waves emanating from the lorry. The principle is best represented diagrammatically.

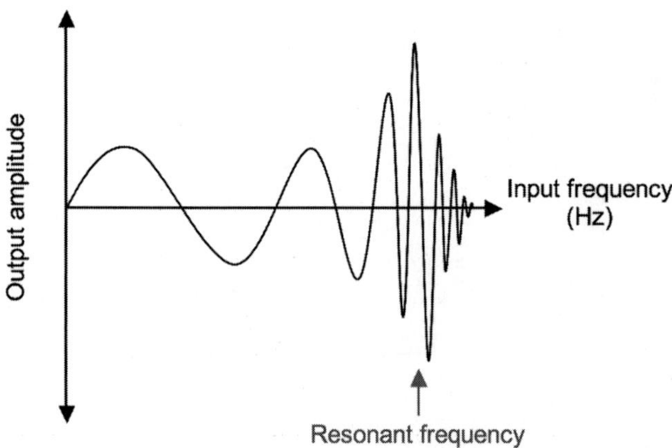

> The curve shows the amplitude of oscillation of an object or system as the frequency of the input oscillation is steadily increased. Start by drawing a normal sine wave whose wavelength decreases as the input frequency increases. Demonstrate a particular frequency at which the amplitude rises to a peak. By no means does this have to occur at a high frequency; it depends on what the natural frequency of the system is. Label the peak amplitude frequency as the resonant frequency. Make sure that, after the peak, the amplitude dies away again towards the baseline.

This subject is most commonly discussed in the context of invasive arterial pressure monitoring.

Damping

> A decrease in the amplitude of an oscillation as a result of energy loss from a system owing to frictional or other resistive forces.

A degree of damping is desirable and necessary for accurate measurement, but too much damping is problematic. The terminology should be considered in the context of a measuring system that is attempting to respond to an instantaneous change in the measured value. This is akin to the situation in which you suddenly stop flushing an arterial line while watching the arterial trace on the theatre monitor.

Damping coefficient

> A value between 0 (no damping) and 1 (critical damping) which quantifies the level of damping present in a system.

Zero damping

> A theoretical situation in which the system oscillates in response to a step change in the input value and the amplitude of the oscillations does not diminish with time; the damping coefficient is 0.

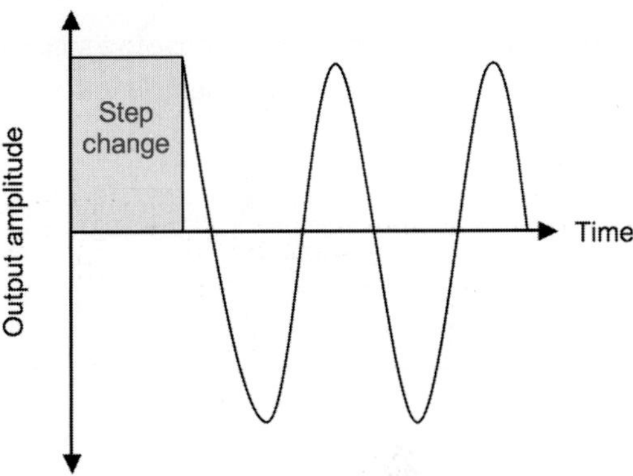

The step change in input value from positive down to baseline initiates a change in the output reading. The system is un-damped because the output value continues to oscillate around the baseline after the input value has changed. The amplitude of these oscillations would remain constant, as shown, if no energy was lost to the surroundings. This situation is, therefore, theoretical as energy is inevitably lost, even in optimal conditions such as a vacuum.

Under-damped

The system is unable to prevent oscillations in response to a step change in the input value. The damping coefficient is 0–0.3.

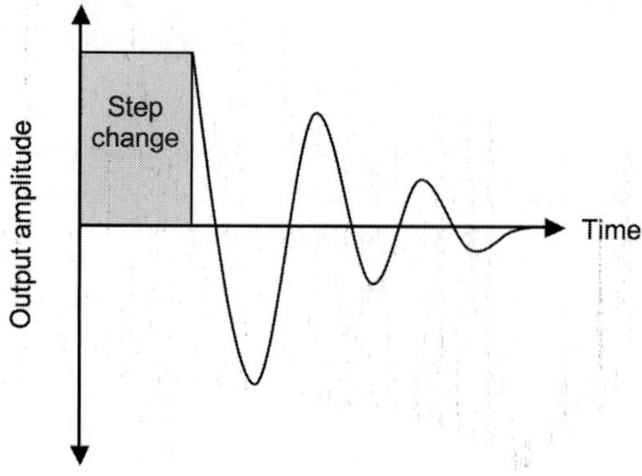

The step change in input value from positive to baseline initiates a change in the output reading. The system is under-damped because the output value continues to oscillate around the baseline for some time after the input value has changed. It does eventually settle at the new value, showing that at least some damping is occurring.

Over-damped

The system response is overly blunted in response to a step change in the input value, leading to inaccuracy. The damping coefficient is > 1.

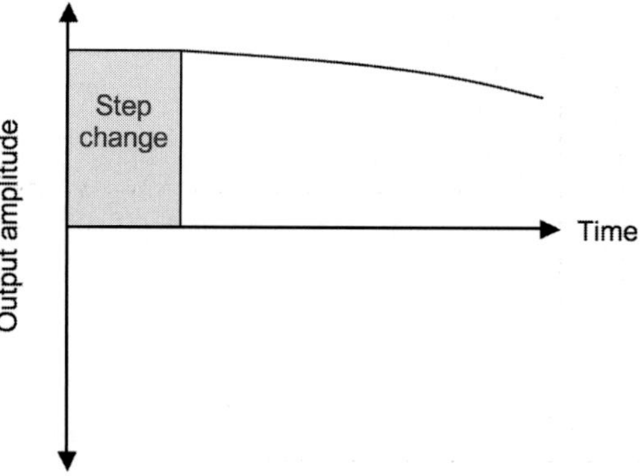

This time the curve falls extremely slowly towards the new value. Given enough time, it will reach the baseline with no overshoot but clearly this type of response is unsuitable for measurement of a rapidly changing variable such as blood pressure.

Critical damping

That degree of damping which allows the most rapid attainment of a new input value combined with no overshoot in the measured response. The damping coefficient is 1.

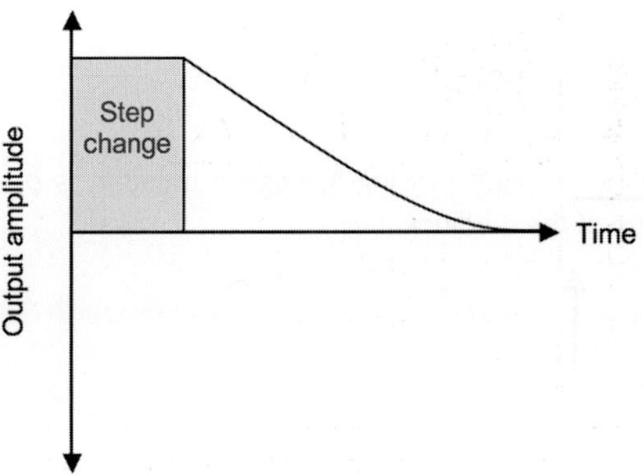

The response is still blunted but any faster response would involve overshoot of the baseline. Critical damping is still too much for a rapidly responding measurement device.

Optimal damping

The most suitable combination of rapid response to change in the input value with minimal overshoot. The damping coefficient is 0.64.

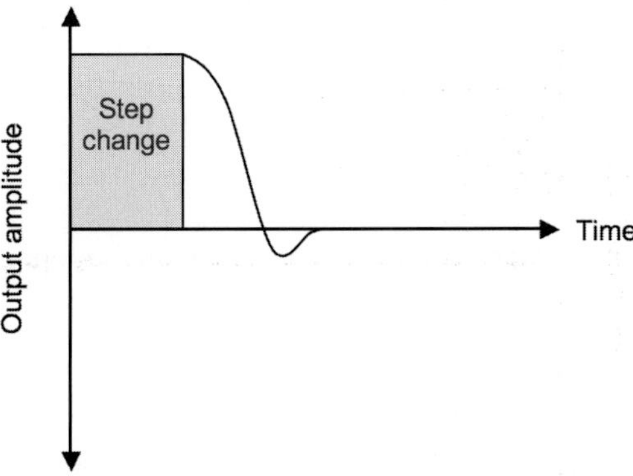

Draw this curve so that the response is fairly rapid with no more than two oscillations around the baseline before attaining the new value. This is the level of damping that is desirable in modern measuring systems.

Pulse oximetry

There are a number of equations and definitions associated with the principles behind the working of the pulse oximeter.

Beer's law

The absorbance of light passing through a medium is proportional to the concentration of the medium.

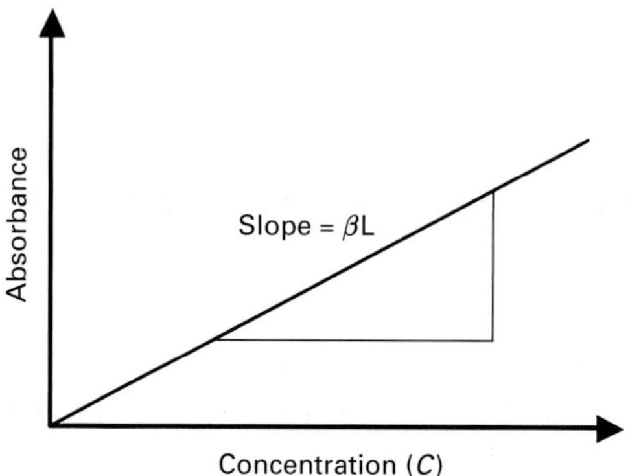

Draw a line that passes through the origin and which rises steadily as C increases. The slope of the line is dependent upon the molar extinction coefficient (β), which is a measure of how avidly the medium absorbs light, and by the path length (L). Note that if emergent light (I) is plotted on the y axis instead of absorbance, the curve should be drawn as an exponential decline.

Lambert's law

The absorbance of light passing through a medium is proportional to the path length.

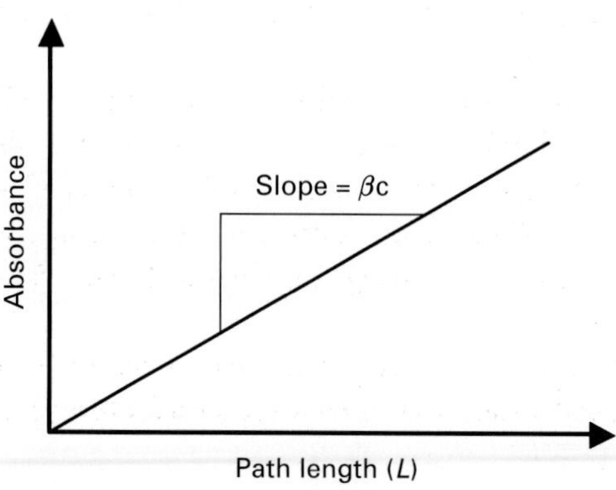

The line is identical to that above except that in this instance the slope is determined by both β and the concentration (C) of the medium. Again, if emergent light (I) is plotted on the y axis instead of absorbance, the curve should be plotted as an exponential decline.

Both laws are often presented together to give the following equation, known as the **Beer–Lambert law**, which is a negative exponential equation of the form $y = a.e^{-kt}$

$$I = I_0.e^{-(LC\beta)}$$

or taking logarithms

$$log(I_0/I) = LC\beta$$

where I is emergent light, I_0 is incident light, L is path length, C is concentration and β is the molar extinction coefficient.

The relation $\log(I_0/I)$ is known as the **absorbance**.

In the pulse oximeter, the concentration and molar extinction coefficient are constant. The only variable becomes the path length, which alters as arterial blood expands the vessels in a pulsatile fashion.

Haemoglobin absorption spectra

The pulse oximeter is a non-invasive device used to monitor the percentage saturation of haemoglobin (Hb) with oxygen (Spo_2). The underlying physical principle that allows this calculation to take place is that infrared light is absorbed to different degrees by the oxy and deoxy forms of Hb.

Two different wavelengths of light, one at 660 nm (red) and one at 940 nm (infrared), are shone intermittently through the finger to a sensor. As the vessels in the finger expand and contract with the pulse, they alter the amount of light that is absorbed at each wavelength according to the Beer–Lambert law. The pulsatile vessels, therefore, cause two waveforms to be produced by the sensor.

If there is an excess of deoxy-Hb present, more red than infrared light will be absorbed and the amplitude of the 'red' waveform will be smaller. Conversely, if there is an excess of oxy-Hb, the amplitude of the 'infrared' waveform will be smaller. It is the ratios of these amplitudes that allows the microprocessor to give an estimate of the Spo_2 by comparing the values with those from tables stored in its memory.

In order to calculate the amount of oxy-Hb or deoxy-Hb present from the amount of light absorbance, the absorbance spectra for these compounds must be known.

Haemoglobin absorption spectra

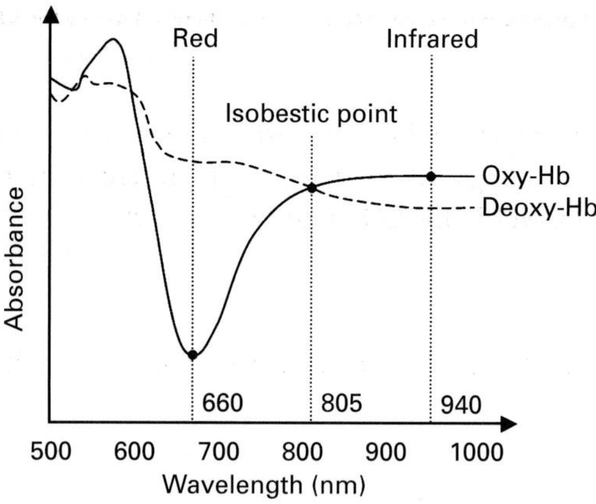

Oxy-Hb Crosses the *y* axis near the deoxy-Hb line but falls steeply around 600 nm to a trough around 660 nm. It then rises as a smooth curve through the isobestic point where it flattens out. This curve must be oxy-Hb as the absorbance of red light is so low that most of it is able to pass through to the viewer, which is why oxygenated blood appears red.

Deoxy-Hb Starts near the oxy-Hb line and falls as a relatively smooth curve passing through the isobestic point only. Compared with oxy-Hb, it absorbs a vast amount of red light and so appears 'blue' to the observer.

Capnography

You will be expected to be familiar with capnography. The points to understand are the shape and meaning of different capnograph traces and the nature of the reaction taking place within the CO_2 absorption canister.

Capnometer

The capnometer measures the partial pressure of CO_2 in a gas and displays the result in numerical form.

Capnograph

A capnograph measures the partial pressure of CO_2 in a gas and displays the result in graphical form.

A capnometer alone is unhelpful in clinical practice and most modern machines present both a graphical and numerical representation of CO_2 partial pressure.

Normal capnograph

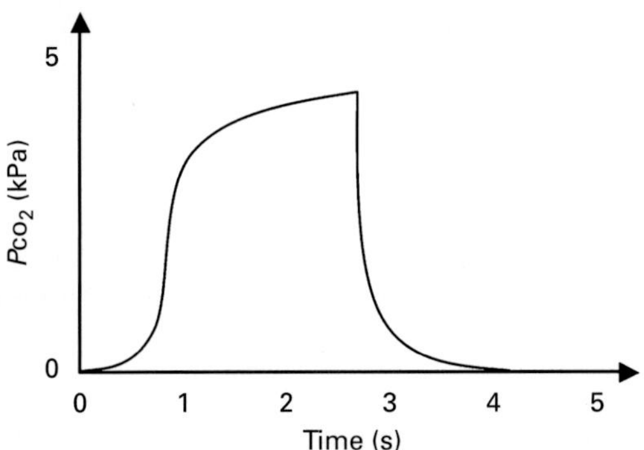

Assume a respiratory rate of 12 min^{-1}. From zero baseline, the curve initially rises slowly owing to the exhalation of dead space gas. Subsequently, it rises steeply during expiration to a normal value and reaches a near horizontal plateau after approximately 3 s. The value just prior to inspiration is the end-tidal CO_2 (P_{ETCO_2}) . Inspiration causes a near vertical decline in the curve to baseline and lasts around 2 s.

Rebreathing

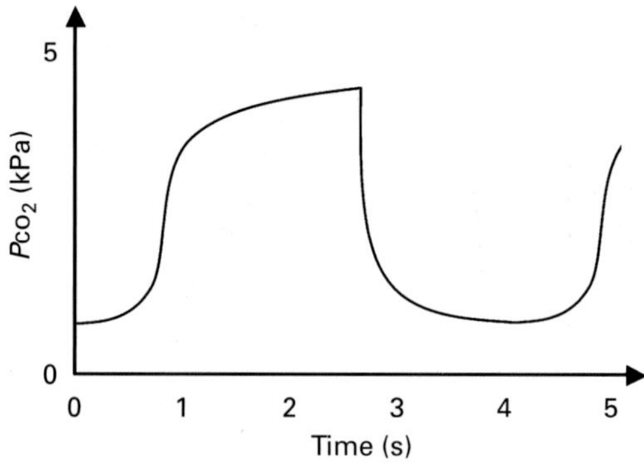

The main difference when compared rebreathing with the normal trace is that the baseline is not zero. Consequently the P_{ETCO_2} may rise. If the patient is spontaneously breathing, the respiratory rate may increase as they attempt to compensate for the higher P_{ETCO_2}.

Inadequate paralysis

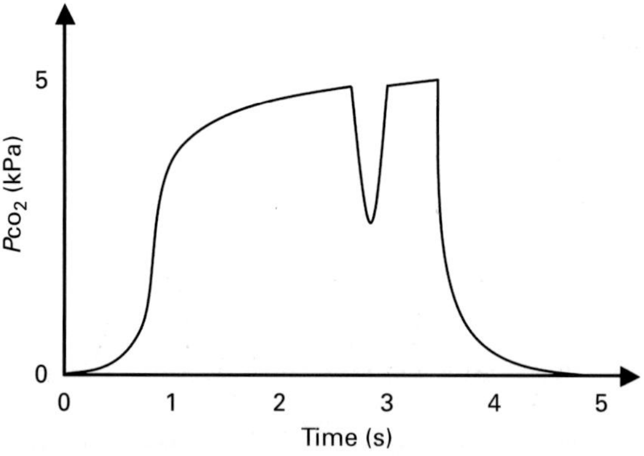

The bulk of the curve appears identical to the normal curve. However, during the plateau phase, a large cleft is seen as the patient makes a transient respiratory effort and draws fresh gas over the sensor.

Cardiac oscillations

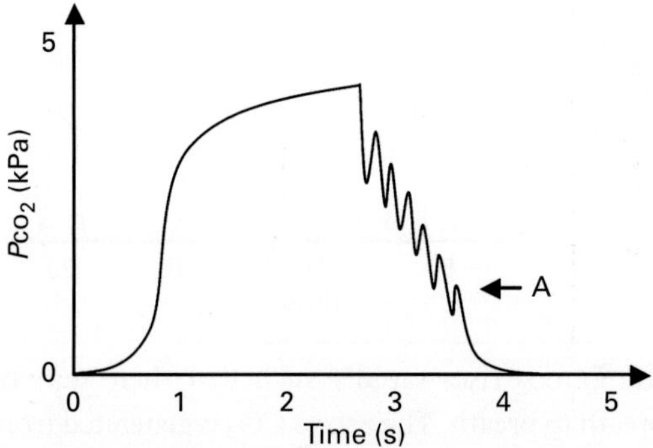

Usually seen when the respiratory rate is slow. The curve starts as normal but the expiratory pause is prolonged owing to the slow rate. Fresh gas within the circuit is able to pass over the sensor causing the $P\text{CO}_2$ to fall. During this time, the mechanical pulsations induced by the heart force small quantities of alveolar gas out of the lungs and over the sensor, causing transient spikes. Inspiration in the above example does not occur until point A.

Hyperventilation

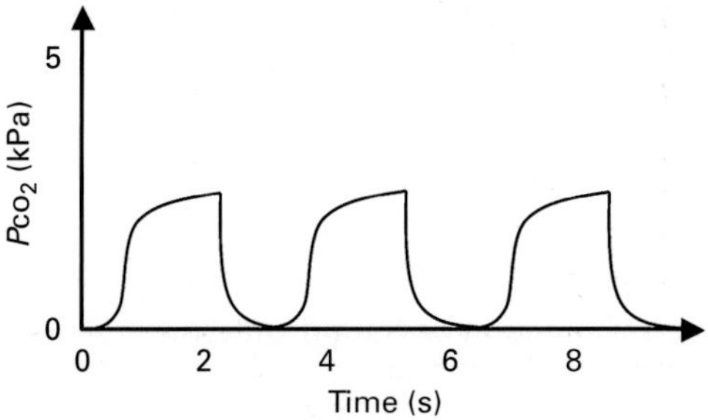

In this example, the respiratory rate has increased so that each respiratory cycle only takes 3 s. As a consequence the P_{ETCO_2} has fallen to approx 2.5 kPa.

Malignant hyperpyrexia

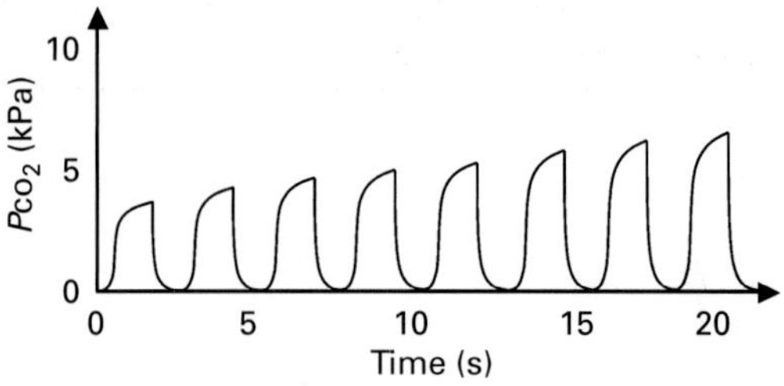

Rarely seen. The P_{ETCO_2} rises rapidly such that there may be a noticeable increase from breath to breath. The excess CO_2 is generated from the increased skeletal muscle activity and metabolic rate, which is a feature of the condition.

Acute loss of cardiac output

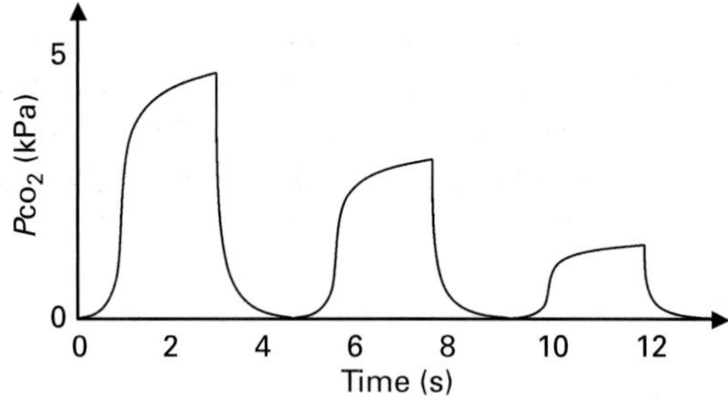

The P_{ETCO_2} falls rapidly over the course of a few breaths. With hyperventilation, the fall would be slower. Any condition that acutely reduces cardiac output may be the cause, including cardiac arrest, pulmonary embolism or acute rhythm disturbances. If the P_{CO_2} falls *instantly* to zero, then the cause is disconnection, auto-calibration or equipment error.

Breathing system disconnection

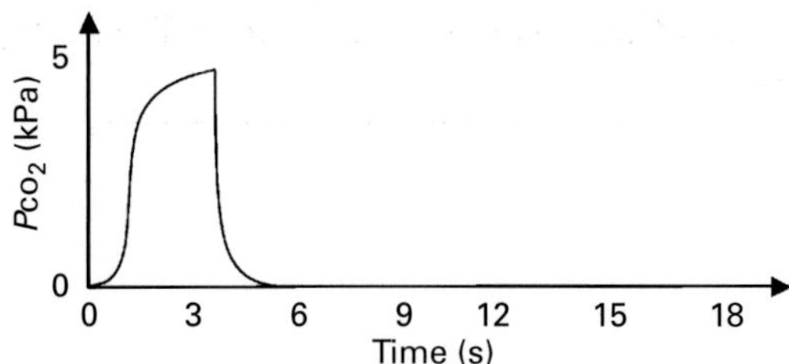

Following a normal trace, there is the absence of any further rise in $P\text{CO}_2$. You should ensure that your x axis is long enough to demonstrate that this is not simply a result of a slow respiratory rate.

Obstructive disease

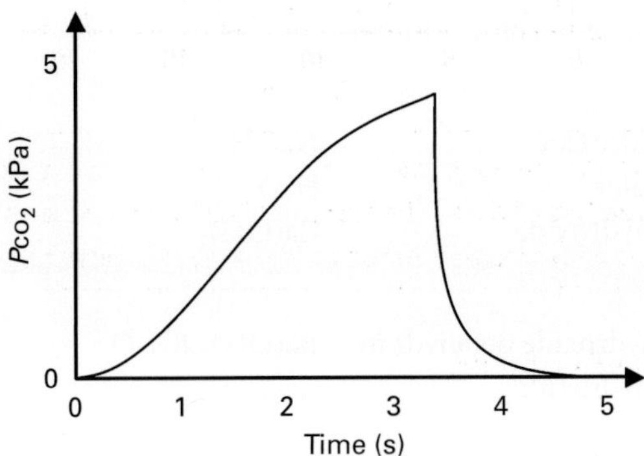

Instead of the normal sharp upstroke, the curve should be drawn slurred. This occurs because lung units tend to empty slowly in obstructive airways disease. In addition, the $P\text{ETCO}_2$ may be raised as a feature of the underlying disease.

Hypoventilation

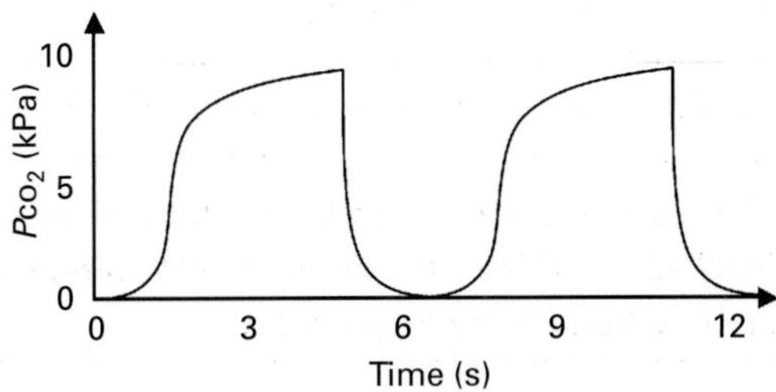

The respiratory rate is reduced such that each complete respiratory cycle takes longer. This is usually a result of a prolonged expiratory phase, so it is the plateau that you should demonstrate to be extended. The $P\text{ETCO}_2$ will be raised as a consequence.

Absorption of carbon dioxide

Carbon dioxide is absorbed in most anaesthetic breathing systems by means of a canister that contains a specific absorbing medium. This is often soda lime but may also be baralime in some hospitals.

Soda lime:

4% sodium hydroxide	$NaOH$
15% bound water	H_2O
81% calcium hydroxide	$Ca(OH)_2$

Baralime:

20% barium hydroxide octahydrate	$Ba(OH)_2.8H_2O$
80% calcium hydroxide	$Ca(OH)_2$

Mesh size

The smaller the granules, the larger the surface area for CO_2 absorption. However, if the granules are too small then there will be too little space between them and the resistance to gas flow through the canister will be too high. As a compromise, a 4/8 mesh describes the situation where each granule should be able to pass through a sieve with four openings per inch but not through one with eight openings per inch.

Chemical reaction

You may be asked to describe the chemical reaction that occurs when CO_2 is absorbed within the canister. The most commonly cited reaction is that between soda lime and CO_2:

$$CO_2 + H_2O \rightarrow H_2CO_3$$
$$2NaOH + H_2CO_3 \rightarrow Na_2CO_3 + 2H_2O + \text{heat}$$
$$Na_2CO_3 + Ca(OH)_2 \rightarrow CaCO_3 + 2NaOH + \text{heat}$$

Heat is produced at two stages and water at one. This can be seen and felt in clinical practice. Note that NaOH is reformed in the final stage and so acts only as a catalyst for the reaction. The compound that is actually consumed in both baralime and soda lime is $Ca(OH)_2$.

Colour indicators

Compound	Colour change
Ethyl violet	White to purple
Clayton yellow	Pink to cream
Titan yellow	Pink to cream
Mimosa Z	Red to white
Phenolphthalein	Red to white

Cardiac output measurement

The Fick principle

The total uptake or release of a substance by an organ is equal to the product of the blood flow to the organ and the arterio-venous concentration difference of the substance.

This observation is used to calculate cardiac output by using a suitable marker substance such as oxygen, heat or dye and the following equation:

$$\dot{V}O_2 = CO\ (CaO_2 - C\bar{v}O_2)$$

so

$$CO = \dot{V}O_2/(CaO_2 - C\bar{v}O_2)$$

where $\dot{V}O_2$ is the oxygen uptake, CO is cardiac output, CaO_2 is arterial O_2 content and $C\bar{v}O_2$ is mixed venous O_2 content.

Thermodilution and dye dilution

A marker substance is injected into a central vein. A peripheral arterial line is used to measure the amount of the substance in the arterial system. A graph of concentration versus time is produced and patented algorithms based on the Stewart–Hamilton equation (below) are used to calculate the cardiac output.

When dye dilution is used, the graph of concentration versus time may show a second peak as dye recirculates to the measuring device. This is known as a recirculation hump and does not occur when thermodilution methods are used.

Stewart–Hamilton equation

If the mass of marker is known and its concentration is measured, the volume into which it was given can be calculated as

$$V = M/C$$

If concentration is measured over time, flow can be calculated as

$$\text{Flow} = M/(C.\Delta t)$$

where M is mass, V is volume and C is concentration. A special form of the equation used with thermodilution is

$$\text{Flow} = \frac{V_{\text{inj}}(T_{\text{b}} - T_{\text{t}}).K}{T_{\text{blood}}(t)t}$$

where the numerator represents the 'mass' of cold and the denominator represents the change in blood temperature over time; K represents computer constants.

Dye dilution graphs

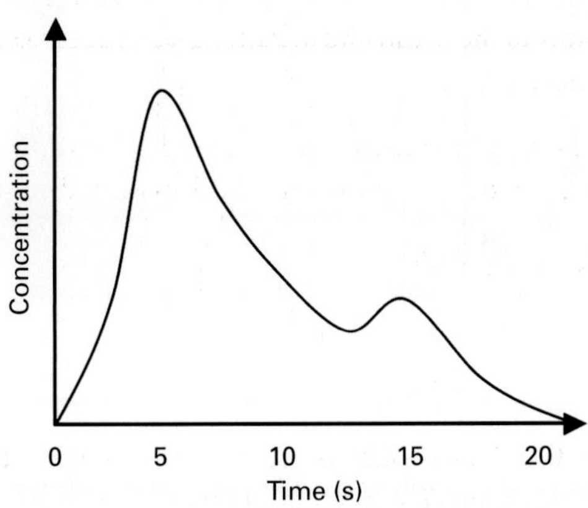

Draw a curve starting at the origin that reaches its maximum value at around 5 s. The curve then falls to baseline but is interrupted by a recirculation hump at around 15 s. This is caused by dye passing completely around the vasculature and back to the sensor a second time.

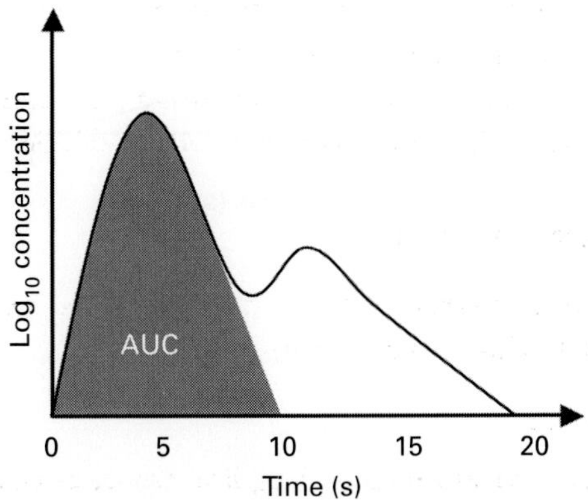

Demonstrate that the semi-log plot makes the curve more linear during its rise and fall from baseline. The recirculation hump is still present but is discounted by measuring the area under the curve (AUC) enclosed by a tangent from the initial down stroke. This is the AUC that is used in the calculations.

Thermodilution graphs

The actual graph of temperature versus time for the thermodilution method would resemble the one below.

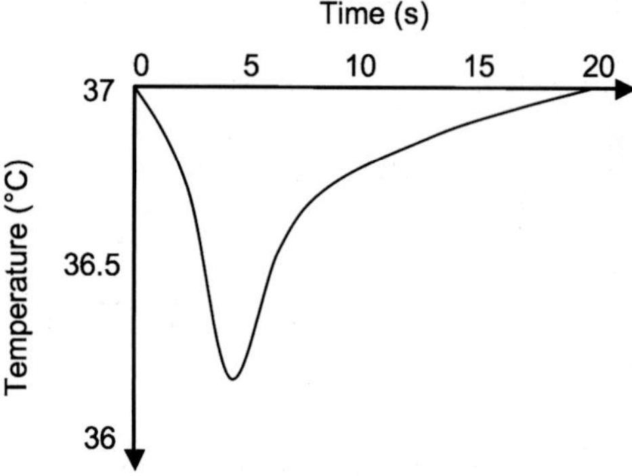

Demonstrate that the thermodilution curve has no recirculation hump when compared with the dye dilution method. Otherwise the line should be drawn in a similar fashion.

For reasons of clarity, the graph is usually presented with temperature *decrease* on the *y* axis so that the deflection becomes positive.

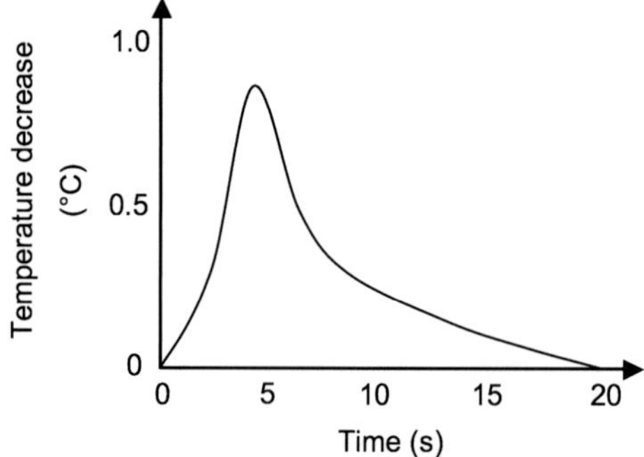

Thermodilution graphs

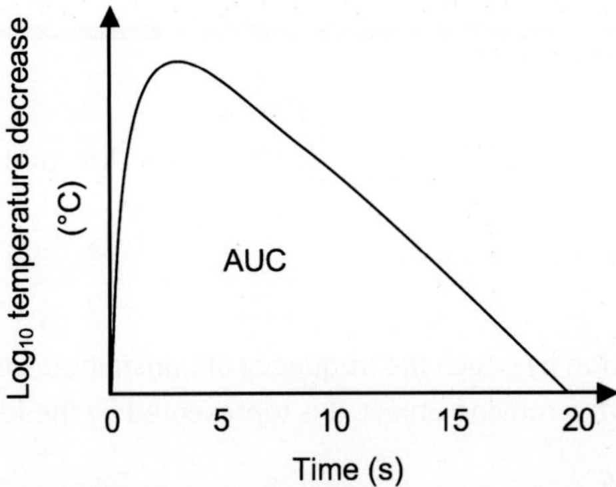

The semi-log transformation again makes the rise and fall of the graph linear. Note that this time there is no recirculation hump. As the fall on the initial plot was exponential, so the curve is transformed to a linear fall by plotting it as a semi-log. The AUC is still used in the calculations of cardiac output.

The Doppler effect

The Doppler effect is used in practice to visualize directional blood flow on ultrasound, to estimate cardiac output and in some types of flow meter.

Doppler effect

The phenomenon by which the frequency of transmitted sound is altered as it is reflected from a moving object. It is represented by the following equation:

$$V = \frac{\Delta F.c}{2F_0.\cos\theta}$$

where V is velocity of object, ΔF is frequency shift, c is speed of sound in blood, F_0 is frequency of emitted sound and θ is the angle between sound and object.

Principle

Sound waves are emitted from the probe (P) at a frequency F_0. They are reflected off moving red blood cells and back towards the probe at a new frequency, F_R. The phase shift can now be determined by $F_R - F_0$. The angle of incidence (θ) is shown on the diagram . If a measurement or estimate of the cross-sectional area of the blood vessel is known, flow can be derived as area multiplied by velocity ($m^2.m.s^{-1} = m^3.s^{-1}$). This is the principle behind oesophageal Doppler cardiac output monitoring.

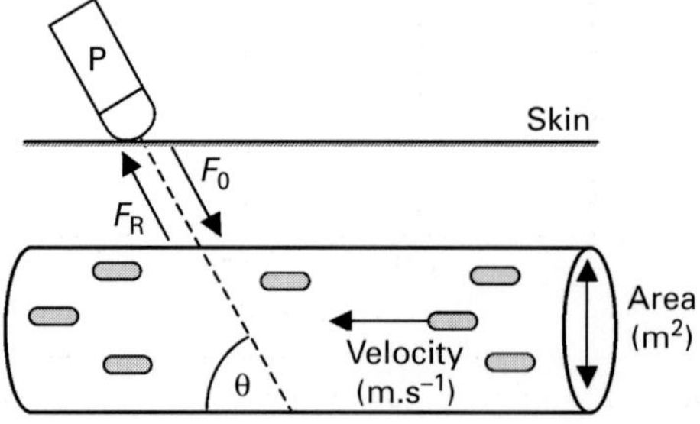

It is also possible to calculate the pressure gradients across heart valves using the Doppler principle to measure the blood velocity and entering the result into the Bernoulli equation.

Bernoulli equation

$$\Delta P = 4v^2$$

where ΔP is the pressure gradient and v is the velocity of blood.

Neuromuscular blockade monitoring

This topic tests your knowledge of the physics and physiology behind the use of neuromuscular blocking drugs (NMBDs). You will benefit from a clear idea in your mind about what each type of nerve stimulation pattern is attempting to demonstrate.

Single twitch

A single, supra-maximal stimulus is applied prior to neuromuscular blockade as a control. The diminution in twitch height and disappearance of the twitch correlates crudely with depth of neuromuscular block.

Supra-maximal stimulus

An electrical stimulus of sufficient current magnitude to depolarize all nerve fibres within a given nerve bundle. Commonly quoted as > 60 mA for transcutaneous nerve stimulation.

Train of four

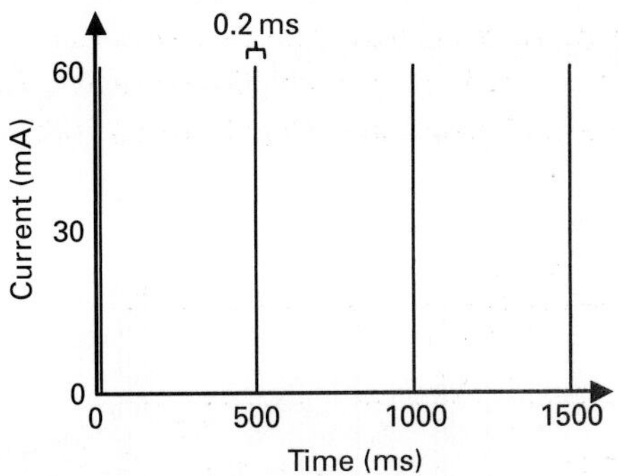

Notice that you are being asked to describe the output waveform of the nerve stimulator. The axes must, therefore, be time and current as shown. Each stimulus is a square wave of supra-maximal current delivered for 0.2 ms. The train of four (TOF) is delivered at 2 Hz so there is one stimulus every 500 ms. This means that if the TOF starts at time 0, the complete train takes 1500 ms.

Tetanic stimulus

A supra-maximal stimulus applied as a series of square waves of 0.2 ms duration at a frequency of 50 Hz for a duration of 5 s is tetanic stimulation.

Depolarizing block train of four

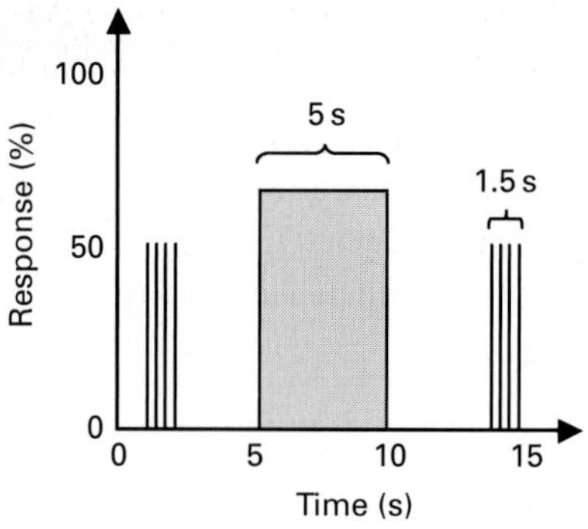

Notice now that you are being asked to describe the response to a TOF stimulus. The axes are, therefore, changed to show time and percentage response as shown. It is important to realize that each twitch is still being delivered at the same current even though the response seen may be reduced. Partial depolarizing neuromuscular block causes an equal decrease in the percentage response to all four stimuli in the TOF. After a period of tetany that does not cause 100% response, there is no increase in the height of subsequent twitches.

Non-depolarizing block train of four

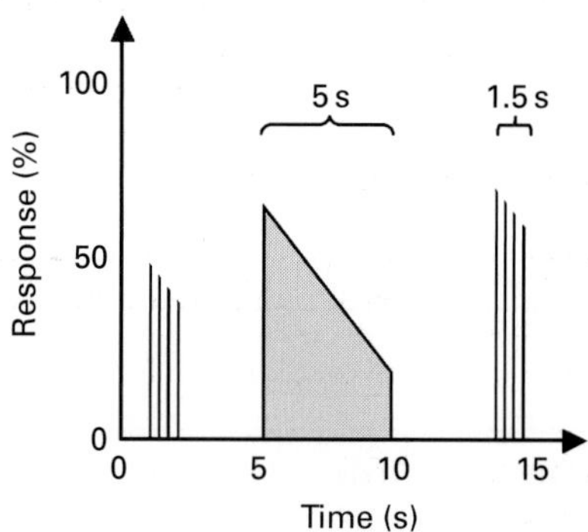

Initial TOF should demonstrate each successive twitch decreasing in amplitude: this is fade. The tetanic stimulus should fail to reach 100% response and should also demonstrate fade. The second TOF should still demonstrate fade but the twitches as a group should have increased amplitude. This is post-tetanic potentiation.

Train of four ratio

The ratio of the amplitudes of the fourth to the first twitches of a TOF stimulus is known as the TOF ratio (TOFR); it is usually given as a percentage T4:T1.

The TOFR is used for assessing suitability for and adequacy of reversal. Three twitches should be present before a reversal agent is administered and the TOFR after reversal should be > 90% to ensure adequacy.

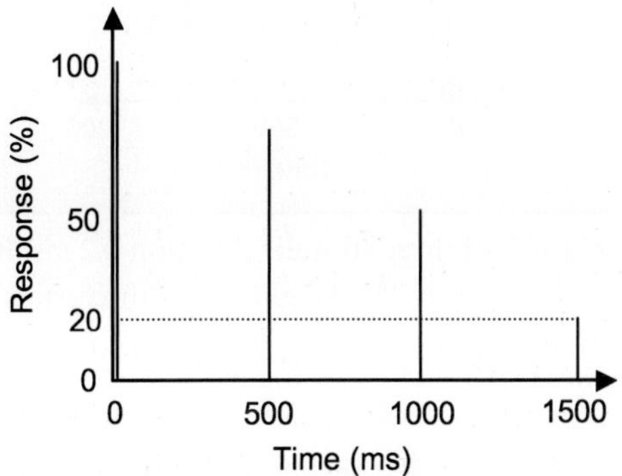

Draw four twitches at 0.5 s intervals with each being lesser in amplitude than its predecessor. In the example, the TOFR is 20% as T4 gives 20% of the response of T1. Explain that this patient would be suitable for reversal as all four twitches are present. However, had this trace been elicited after the administration of a reversal agent, the pattern would represent an inadequate level of reversal for extubation (TOFR < 90%).

Assessment of receptor site occupancy

Twitches seen	Percentage receptor sites blocked
All present	< 70
1 twitch lost	> 70
2 twitches lost	> 80
3 twitches lost	> 90
All lost	95–100

Double-burst stimulation

Two bursts of three stimuli at 50 Hz, each burst being separated by 750 ms.

In double-burst stimulation, the ratio of the second to the first twitch is assessed. There are the same requirements for adequacy of reversal as TOFR (>90%); however, having only two visible twitches makes assessment of the ratio easier for the observer.

No neuromuscular block

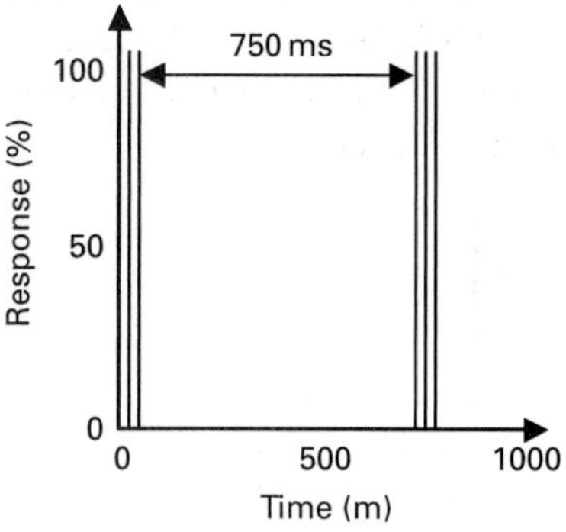

Demonstrate two clusters of three stimuli (duration 0.2 ms, frequency 50 Hz) separated by a 750 ms interval. The heights of both clusters are identical. If questioned, the current should be greater than 60 mA for the same reasons as when using the TOF.

Residual neuromuscular block

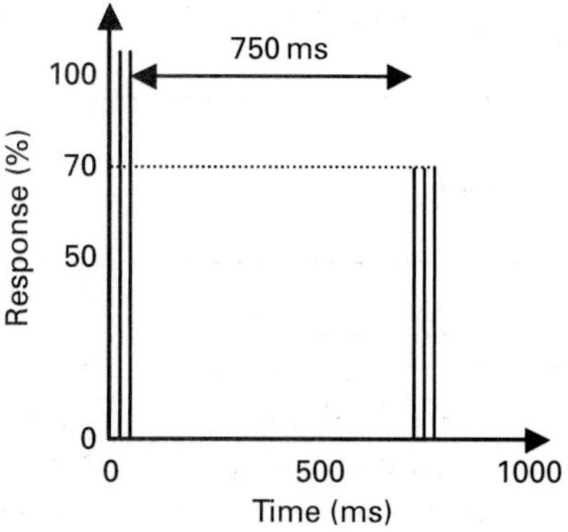

Demonstrate the two clusters with the same time separation. In the presence of a neuromuscular blocking agent, the second cluster will have a lesser amplitude than the first (70% is shown).

Post-tetanic count

A post-tetanic count is used predominantly where neuromuscular blockade is so deep that there are no visible twitches on TOF. The post-tetanic twitch count can help to estimate the likely time to recovery of the TOF twitches in these situations. The meaning of the count is drug specific.

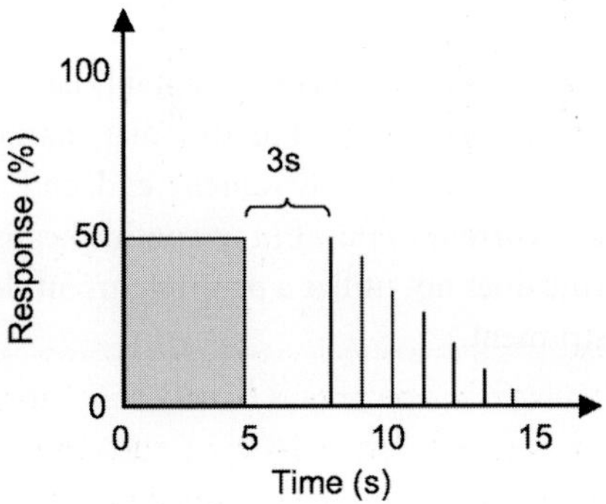

Draw a 5 s period of tetany followed by a 3 s pause. Note that the tetanic stimulus fails to reach 100% response as this test is being used in cases of profound muscle relaxation. Next draw single standard twitches at a frequency of 1 Hz: 20 stimuli are given in total. Using atracurium, a single twitch on the TOF should appear in approximately 4 min if there are four post-tetanic twitches evident.

Phase 1 and phase 2 block

	Phase 1	Phase 2
Cause	Single dose of depolarizing muscle relaxant	Repeated doses of depolarizing muscle relaxant
Nature of block	Partial depolarizing	Partial non-depolarizing
Single twitch	Decreased	Decreased
T4:T1	> 0.7	< 0.7
1 Hz twitch	Sustained	Fade
Post-tetanic potentiation	No	Yes
Effect of anticholinesterases	Block augmented	Block antagonized

Surgical diathermy

The principle behind the use of surgical diathermy is that of current density. When a current is applied over a small area, the current density is high and heating may occur. If the same current is applied over a suitably large area then the current density is low and no heating occurs. For unipolar diathermy, the apparatus utilizes a small surface area at the instrument end and a large area on the diathermy plate to allow current to flow but to confine heating to the instrument alone. Bipolar diathermy does not utilize a plate as current flows directly between two points on the instrument.

Frequency

The safety of diathermy is enhanced by the use of high frequency (1 MHz) current, as explained by the graph below.

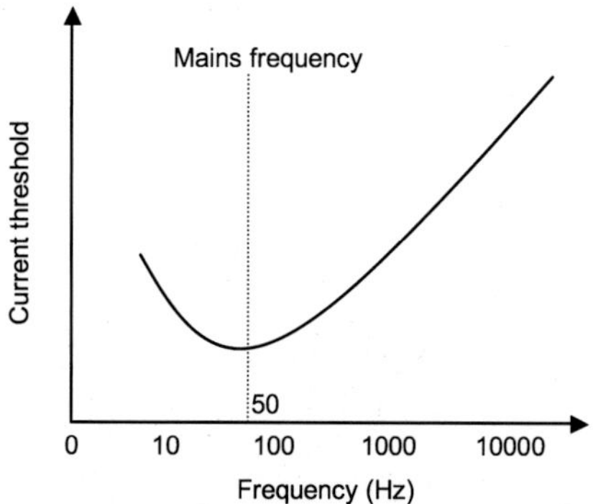

Note that the *x* axis is logarithmic to allow a wide range of frequencies to be shown. The *y* axis is the current threshold at which adverse physiological events (dysrhythmias etc.) may occur. The highest risk of an adverse event occurs at current frequencies of around 50 Hz, which is the UK mains frequency. At diathermy frequencies, the threshold for an adverse event is massively raised.

Cutting diathermy

This type of diathermy is used to cut tissues and is high energy. It differs from coagulation diathermy by its waveform.

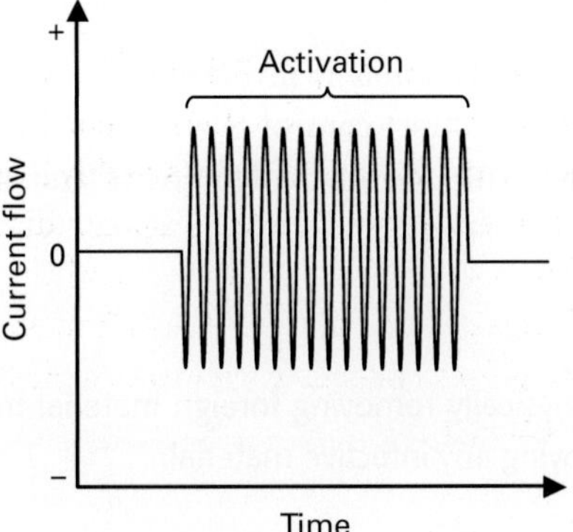

When activated, the instrument delivers a sustained high-frequency AC waveform. Current density is high at the implement and local heating causes tissue destruction. The sine wave continues until the switch is released.

Coagulation diathermy

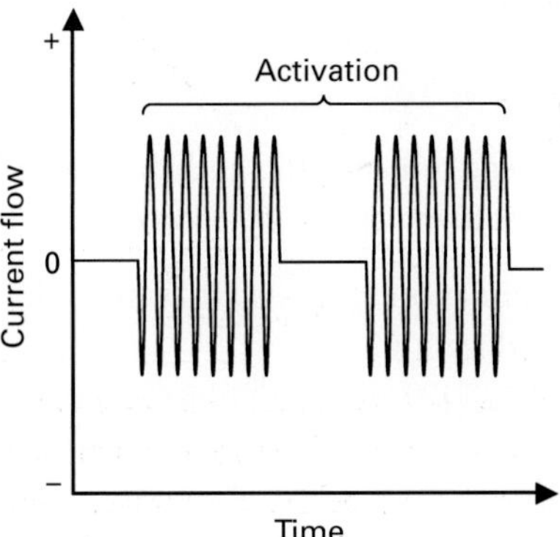

When activated, the instrument delivers bursts of high-frequency AC interrupted by periods of no current flow. Local tissue heating still occurs but is not sustained and, therefore, causes less destruction than cutting diathermy.

Cleaning, disinfection and sterilization

Maintaining cleanliness and sterility is involved in everyday practice but, for the most part, is not under the direct control of anaesthetists. Nevertheless, a familiarity will be expected with the main definitions and methods of achieving adequate cleanliness.

Cleaning

The process of physically removing foreign material from an object without necessarily destroying any infective material.

Disinfection

The process of rendering an object free from all pathogenic organisms except bacterial spores.

Sterilization

The process of rendering an object completely free of all viable infectious agents including bacterial spores.

Decontamination

The process of removing contaminants such that they are unable to reach a site in sufficient quantities to initiate an infection or other harmful reaction.

The process of decontamination always starts with cleaning and is followed by either disinfection or sterilization.

Methods

	Technique	Process
Cleaning	Manual	Washing
	Automated	Ultrasonic bath
	Automated	Low-temperature steam
Disinfection	Chemical	Gluteraldehyde 2%
	Chemical	Alcohol 60–80%
	Chemical	Chlorhexidine 0.5–5%
	Chemical	Hydrogen peroxide
	Heat	Pasteurization
Sterilization	Chemical	Ethylene oxide
	Chemical	Gluteraldehyde 2%
	Heat	Autoclave
	Radiation	Gamma irradiation
	Other	Gas plasma

The Meyer–Overton hypothesis

The Meyer–Overton hypothesis is the theory of anaesthetic action which proposes that the potency of an anaesthetic agent is related to its lipid solubility.

Potency is described by the minimum alveolar concentration (MAC) of an agent and lipid solubility by the oil:gas solubility coefficient.

Minimum alveolar concentration

The minimum alveolar concentration of an anaesthetic vapour at equilibrium is the concentration required to prevent movement to a standardized surgical stimulus in 50% of unpremedicated subjects studied at sea level (1 atmosphere).

The Meyer–Overton hypothesis proposed that once a sufficient number of anaesthetic molecules were dissolved in the lipid membranes of cells within the central nervous system, anaesthesia would result by a mechanism of membrane disruption. While an interesting observation, there are several exceptions to the rule that make it insufficient to account fully for the mechanism of anaesthesia.

Meyer–Overton graph of potency versus lipid solubility

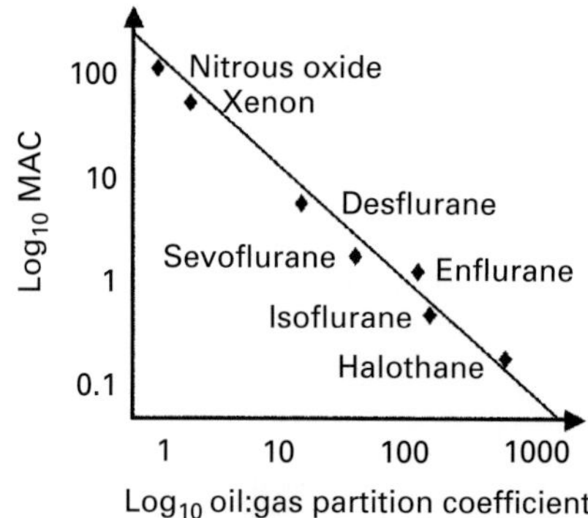

After drawing and labelling the axis (note the slightly different scales), draw a straight line with a negative gradient as shown. Make sure you can draw in the position of the commonly used inhalational agents. Note that the line does not pass directly through the points but is a line of best fit, and also that although isoflurane and enflurane have near identical oil:gas partition coefficients they have different MAC values and, therefore, this relationship is not perfect.

The concentration and second gas effects

The concentration effect

> The phenomenon by which the rise in the alveolar partial pressure of nitrous oxide is disproportionately rapid when it is administered in high concentrations.

Nitrous oxide (N_2O), although relatively insoluble, is 20 times more soluble in the blood than nitrogen (N_2). The outward diffusion of N_2O from the alveolus into the blood is therefore much faster than the inward diffusion of N_2 from the blood into the alveolus. Consequently, the alveolus shrinks in volume and the remaining N_2O is concentrated within it. This smaller volume has a secondary effect of increasing alveolar ventilation by drawing more gas into the alveolus from the airways in order to replenish the reduced volume.

Graphical demonstration

The above concept can be described graphically by considering the fractional concentration of an agent in the alveolar gas (*F*A) as a percentage of its fractional concentration in the inhaled gas (*F*I) over time.

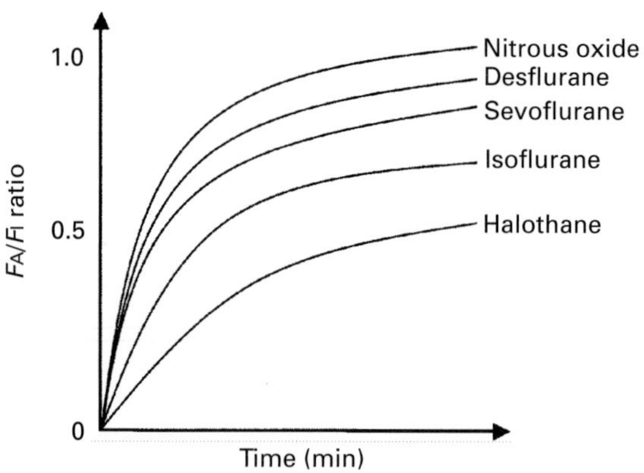

After drawing and labelling the axis draw a series of build-up negative exponential curves with different gradients as shown. The order of the curves is according to the blood:gas partition coefficients. The more insoluble the agent, the steeper the curve and the faster the rate of onset. The exceptions to this are the N_2O and desflurane curves, which are the opposite way round. This is because of the concentration effect when N_2O is administered at high flows and is the graphical representation of the word 'disproportionately' in the definition. You may be asked what would happen as time progressed and you should indicate that the lines eventually form a plateau at an F_A/F_I ratio of 1.0.

The second gas effect

The phenomenon by which the speed of onset of inhalational anaesthetic agents is increased when they are administered with N_2O as a carrier gas.

This occurs as a result of the concentration effect and so it is always useful to describe the concentration effect first, even if being questioned directly on the second gas effect. If there is another gas present in the alveolus, then it too will be concentrated by the relatively rapid uptake of N_2O into the blood.

Isomerism

Isomerism is a subject which can easily become confusing due to the myriad of definitions and nomenclature it involves. Remembering a schematic diagram such as the one below often helps to focus the mind as to where each type of isomer fits.

Isomerism

The phenomenon by which molecules with the same atomic formulae have different structural arrangements.

Isomers are important because the three-dimensional structure of a drug may determine its effects.

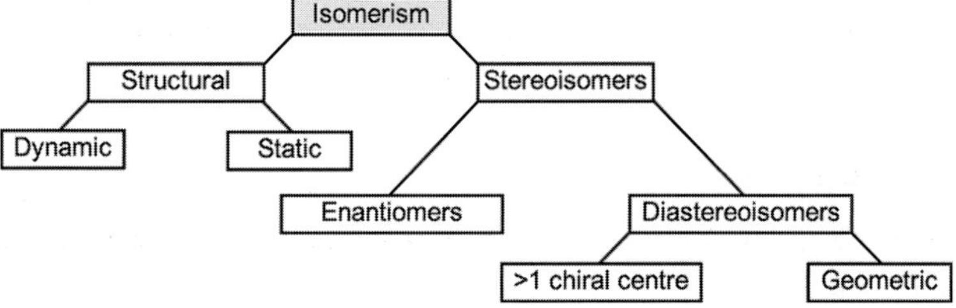

Structural isomerism

Identical chemical formulae but different order of atomic bonds.

Tautomerism

The dynamic interchange between two different forms of a molecular structure depending on the environmental conditions.

Stereoisomerism

Identical chemical formulae and bond structure but different three-dimensional configuration.

Enantiomers

Compounds that have a single chiral centre and form non-superimposable mirror images of each other.

Diastereoisomers

Compounds containing more than one chiral centre or which are subject to geometric isomerism and, therefore, have more than just two mirror image forms.

Geometric isomerism

Two dissimilar groups attached to two atoms that are in turn linked by a double bond or ring creates geometric isomerism because of the reduced mobility of the double bond or ring.

Chiral centre

A central atom bound to four dissimilar groups.

Chiral centres encountered in anaesthetics usually have carbon or quaternary nitrogen as the chiral centre. Any compound which contains more than one chiral centre is termed a diastereoisomer by definition.

Optical isomerism

Differentiation of compounds by their ability to rotate polarized lights in different directions.

Dextro- and laevorotatory

Compounds can be labelled according to the direction in which a molecule of the substance will rotate polarized light. Abbreviated to either *d*- and *l*- or + and −.

D- and L-prefixes

The use of D- and L-prefixes is a nomenclature for orientation of atomic structure of sugar and amino acid molecules. It is a structural definition and is not related to the optical properties.

Rectus and sinister

Molecules at a chiral centre can be labelled according to the direction in which groups of increasing molecular weight are organized around the centre: rectus and sinister, abbreviated to *R* and *S*, depending on whether the direction of increment is clockwise or anti-clockwise, respectively.

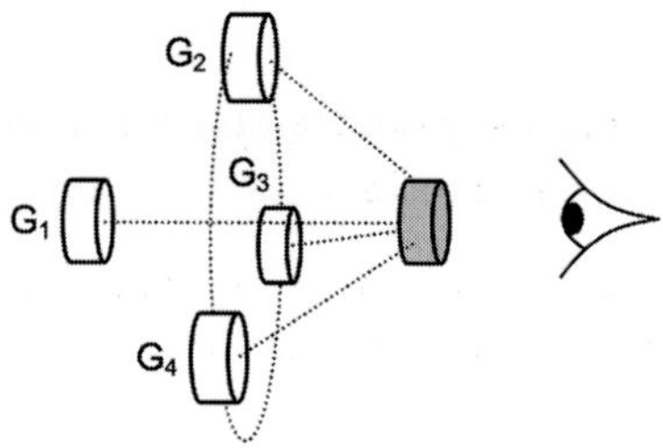

In the diagram, the chiral centre is shaded and attached to four groups of different molecular weights. The smallest group (G_1) is then orientated away from the observer and the remaining groups are assessed. If the groups increase in mass in a clockwise direction as in the figure, the compound is labelled *R*- and vice versa.

Racemic mixture

A mixture of two different enantiomers in equal proportions.

Enantiopure

A preparation with only a single enantiomer present.

Enzyme kinetics

Enzyme

A biological catalyst that increases the speed of a chemical reaction without being consumed in the reaction itself.

The rate of a chemical reaction, therefore, depends on the concentration of the substrates and the presence of the catalysing enzyme.

First-order reaction

A reaction whose rate depends upon the concentration of the reacting components. This is an exponential process.

Zero-order reaction

A reaction whose rate is independent of the concentration of reacting components and is, therefore, constant.

A first-order reaction may become zero order when the enzyme system is saturated.

The Michaelis–Menten equation

Michaelis–Menten equation predicts the rate of a biological reaction according to the concentration of substrate and the specific enzyme characteristics:

$$V = \frac{V_{max}[S]}{K_m + [S]}$$

where V is the velocity of reaction, V_{max} is the maximum velocity of reaction, K_m is the Michaelis constant and [S] is the concentration of substrate.

The value of K_m is the substrate concentration at which $V = ½V_{max}$ and is specific to the particular reaction in question. It is the equivalent of the ED_{50} seen in dose–response curves. This equation has a number of important features.

If [S] is very low, the equation approximates to

$$V \approx \frac{V_{max}[S]}{K_m}$$

as the + [S] term becomes negligible. This means that V is proportional to [S] by a constant of V_{max}/K_m. In other words the reaction is first order.

If [S] is very high the equation approximates to

$$V \approx V_{max}$$

and the reaction becomes zero order, as V is now independent of [S].

Michaelis–Menten graph

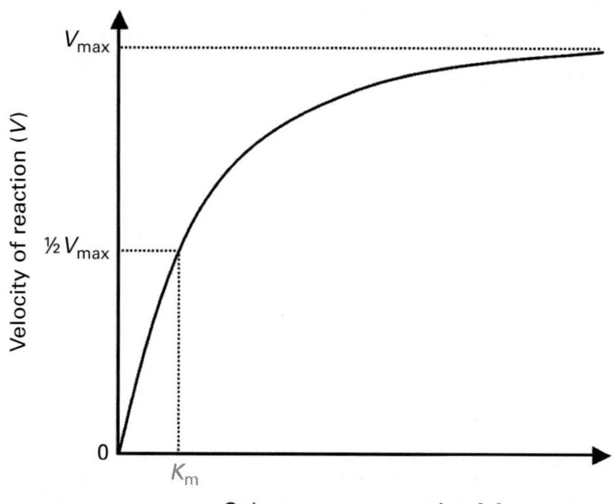

The shape of the curve is an inverted rectangular hyperbola approaching V_{max}. Ensure you mark K_m on the curve at the correct point. The portion of the curve below K_m on the x axis is where the reaction follows first-order kinetics, as shown by a fairly linear rise in the curve with increasing [S]. The portion of the curve to the far right is where the reaction will follow zero-order kinetics, as shown by the almost horizontal gradient. The portion in between these two extremes demonstrates a mixture of properties.

Lineweaver–Burke transformation

To make it easier to measure K_m mathematically a Lineweaver–Burke transformation can be performed by taking reciprocals of both sides of the initial equation.

$$\frac{1}{V} = \frac{K_m + [S]}{V_{max}[S]}$$

This can be rearranged to give

$$\frac{1}{V} = \frac{K_m}{V_{max}[S]} + \frac{1}{V_{max}}$$

or

$$\frac{1}{V} = \left[\frac{K_m}{V_{max}} \cdot \frac{1}{[S]}\right] + \frac{1}{V_{max}}$$

The equation may appear complex but is simply a version of the linear equation

$$y = (ax) + b$$

where y is $1/V$, a is K_m/V_{max}, x is $1/[S]$ and b is $1/V_{max}$.

Lineweaver–Burke graph

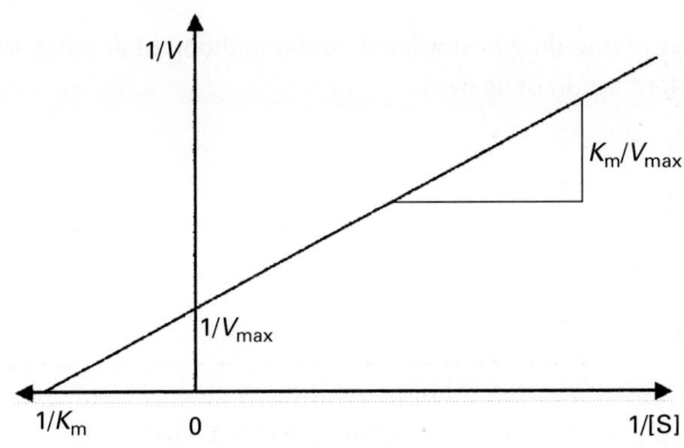

It may help to write the equation down first to remind yourself which functions go where. The simple point of this diagram is that it linearizes the Michaelis–Menten graph and so makes calculation of V_{max} and K_m much easier as they can be found simply by noting the points where the line crosses the y and x axes, respectively, and then taking the inverse value.

Drug interactions

Summation

The actions of two drugs are additive but each has an independent action of its own.

Potentiation

The action of one drug is amplified by the addition of another, which has no independent action of its own.

Synergism

The combined action of two drugs is greater than would be expected from a purely additive effect.

Isobologram

The isobologram shows the amount of drug B that is needed in the face of increasing amounts of drug A in order that the end effect remains constant.

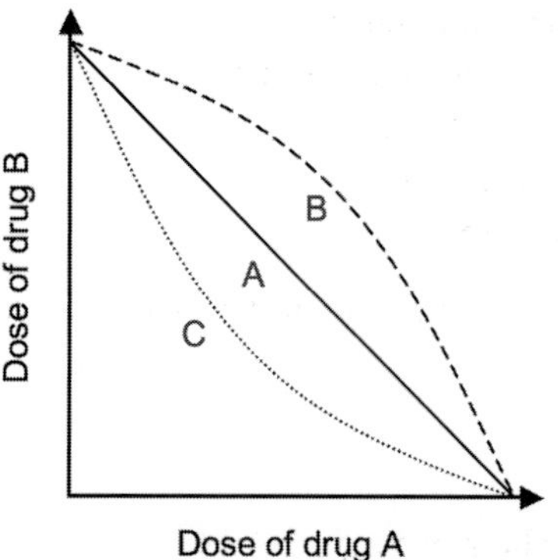

A, additive Draw the axes as shown and a linear relationship labelled A. This represents an additive effect of drug A and drug B such that less of drug B is needed as the dose of drug A is increased.

B, inhibitory Draw an upwardly convex curve labelled B which begins and terminates at the same points as line A. This represents inhibition because now, at any given dose of drug A, more of drug B needs to be given to maintain a constant effect compared with an additive relationship.

C, synergistic Finally draw a downwardly convex curve labelled C. This represents synergy in that less of drug B is required at any point compared with what would be seen with an additive relationship.

Adverse drug reactions

Although not often tested in depth, a knowledge of the terminology used to describe adverse drug reactions is useful. True anaphylactic and anaphylactoid reactions clearly require a more detailed knowledge. The official World Health Organization (WHO) definition of an adverse drug reaction is lengthy and unlikely to be tested. A more succinct definition is used in relation to anaesthesia.

Adverse drug reaction

> The occurrence of any drug effect that is not of therapeutic, diagnostic or prophylactic benefit to the patient.

Types of adverse reactions

The WHO definition encompasses six groups, which need not be memorized but which are included for completeness.

Group 1 Dose-related reactions
Group 2 Non-dose-related reactions
Group 3 Dose- and time-related reactions
Group 4 Time-related reactions
Group 5 Withdrawal reactions
Group 6 Treatment failure.

The reactions can be more simply defined as one of two types:
Type A

- dose dependent
- common
- extension of known pharmacological effect.

Type B

- dose independent
- uncommon
- symptoms and signs of drug allergy.

The most important type to the anaesthetist is type B, which encompasses both anaphylactic and anaphylactoid reactions.

Anaphylactic reaction

A response to a substance to which an individual has been previously sensitized via the formation of a specific IgE antibody. It is characterized by the release of vasoactive substances and the presence of systemic symptoms.

Anaphylactoid reactions

A response to a substance that is not mediated by a specific IgE antibody but is characterized by the same release of vasoactive substances and presence of systemic symptoms as an anaphylactic reaction.

Section 4 • Pharmacodynamics

Drug–receptor interaction

A basic understanding of the interaction between drugs and receptors underlies much of what is covered in the examinations.

Ligand

A ligand is a chemical messenger able to bind to a receptor. May be endogenous or exogenous (drugs).

Receptor

A receptor is a component of a cell that interacts selectively with a compound to initiate the biochemical change or cascade that produces the effects of the compound:

$$D + R \leftrightarrow DR$$

where D is drug, R is receptor and DR is drug–receptor complex.

It is assumed that the magnitude of the response is proportional to the concentration of DR (i.e. [DR]).

Law of mass action

The rate of a reaction is proportional to the concentration of the reacting components.

$$[\mathrm{D}] + [\mathrm{R}] \underset{K_\mathrm{b}}{\overset{K_\mathrm{f}}{\leftrightarrow}} [\mathrm{DR}]$$

where K_f is the rate of forward reaction and K_b is the rate of backward reaction.

At equilibrium, the rates of the forward and back reactions will be the same and the equation can be rearranged

$$K_\mathrm{f}[\mathrm{D}][\mathrm{R}] = K_\mathrm{b}[\mathrm{DR}]$$

The affinity constant

The affinity constant, measured in l/mmol, has the symbol K_A where

$$K_A = K_f/K_b$$

and it reflects the strength of drug–receptor binding

The dissociation constant

The dissociation constant, measured in mmol/l, has the symbol K_D where

$$K_D = K_b/K_f$$

and it reflects the tendency for the drug–receptor complex to split into its component drug and receptor.

Often, K_D is described differently given that the law of mass action states that, at equilibrium

$$K_f[D][R] = K_b[DR]$$

or

$$K_b/K_f = [D][R]/[DR]$$

so

$$K_D = \frac{[D][R]}{[DR]}$$

If a drug has a high affinity, the DR form will be favoured at equilibrium, hence the value of [D][R] will be small and that of [DR] will be high. Therefore, the value of K_D will be small. The opposite is true for a drug with low affinity, where the D and R forms will be favoured at equilibrium.

Another way of looking at K_D is to see what occurs when a drug occupies exactly 50% of receptors at equilibrium. In this case, the number of free receptors [R] will equal that of occupied receptors [DR] and so cancel each other out of the equation above, leaving

$$K_D = [D]$$

In other words

K_D is the molar concentration of a drug at which 50% of its receptors are occupied at equilibrium ($mmol.l^{-1}$).

Classical receptor theory suggests that the response seen will be proportional to the percentage of receptors occupied, although this is not always the case.

Affinity, efficacy and potency

Affinity

A measure of how avidly a drug binds to a receptor.

In the laboratory, affinity can be measured as the concentration of a drug that occupies 50% of the available receptors, as suggested by the definition of K_D.

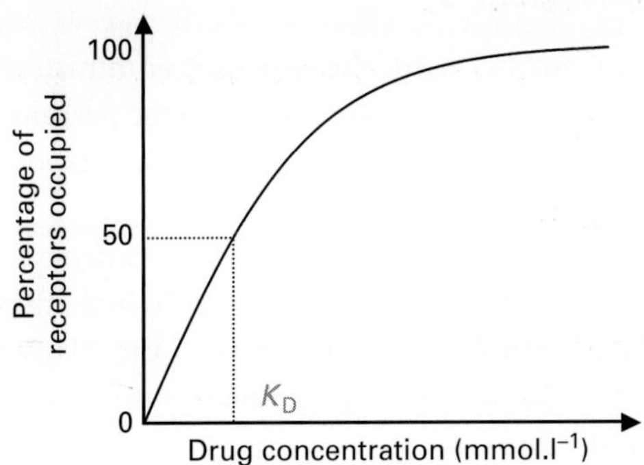

The curve should be drawn as a rectangular hyperbola passing through the origin. K_D is shown and in this situation is a marker of affinity (see text). In practice, drug potency is of more interest, which encompasses both affinity and intrinsic activity. To compare potencies of drugs, the EC_{50} and ED_{50} values (see below) are used.

Efficacy (intrinsic activity)

A measure of the magnitude of the effect once the drug is bound.

Potency

A measure of the quantity of the drug needed to produce maximal effect.

Potency is compared using the **median effective concentration** (EC_{50}) or **median effective dose** (ED_{50}), the meanings of which are subtly different.

Median effective concentration (EC_{50})

The concentration of a drug that induces a specified response exactly half way between baseline and maximum.

This is the measure used in a test where concentration or dose is plotted on the *x* axis and the percentage of maximum response is plotted on the *y* axis. It is a laboratory result of a test performed under a single set of circumstances or on a single animal model.

Median effective dose (ED_{50})

The dose of drug that induces a specified response in 50% of the population to whom it is administered.

This is the measure of potency used when a drug is administered to a population of test subjects. This time the 50% figure refers to the percentage of the *population* responding rather that a percentage of maximal response in a particular individual.

A drug with a lower EC_{50} or ED_{50} will have a higher potency, as it suggests that a lower dose of the drug is needed to produce the desired effect. In practice, the terms are used interchangeably and, of the two, the ED_{50} is the most usual terminology. You are unlikely to get chastised for putting ED_{50} where the correct term should technically be EC_{50}.

Dose–response curves

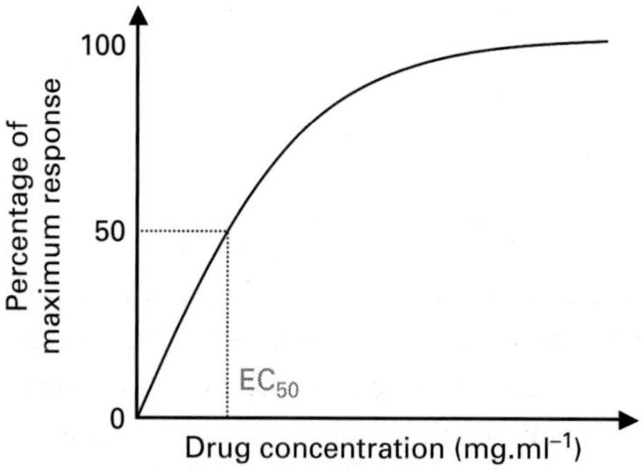

The curve is identical to the first but the axes are labelled differently with percentage of maximum response on the *y* axis. This graph will have been produced from a functional assay in the laboratory on a single subject and is concerned with drug potency. Demonstrate that the EC_{50} is as shown.

Quantal dose–response curves

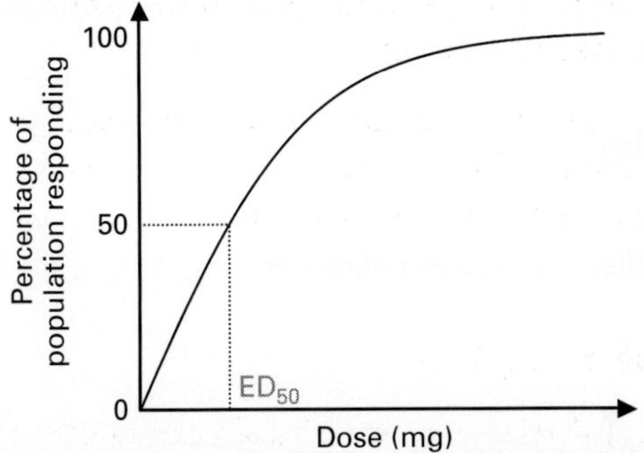

The curve is again identical in shape but this time a population has been studied and the frequency of response recorded at various drug doses. It is, therefore, known as a quantal dose–response curve. The marker of potency is now the ED_{50} and the *y* axis should be correctly labelled as shown. This is the 'typical' dose–response curve that is tested in the examination.

Log dose–response curve

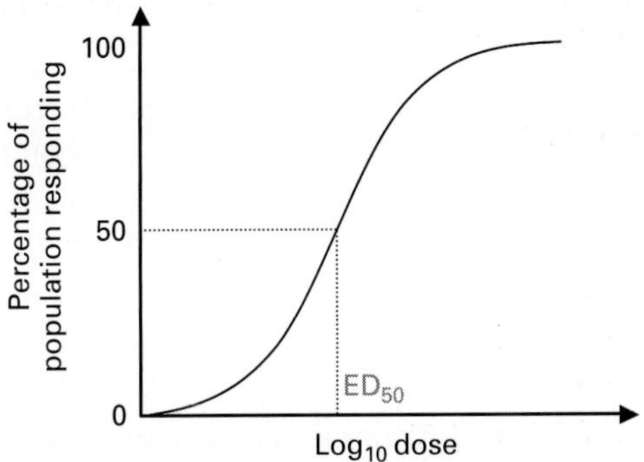

The curve is sigmoid as the *x* axis is now logarithmic. Ensure the middle third of the curve is linear and demonstrate the ED_{50} as shown. Make this your reference curve for a full agonist and use it to compare with other drugs as described below.

Median lethal dose (LD_{50})

The dose of drug that is lethal in 50% of the population to whom it is administered.

Therapeutic index

The therapeutic index of a drug reflects the balance between its useful effects and its toxic effects. It is often defined as

$$LD_{50}/ED_{50}$$

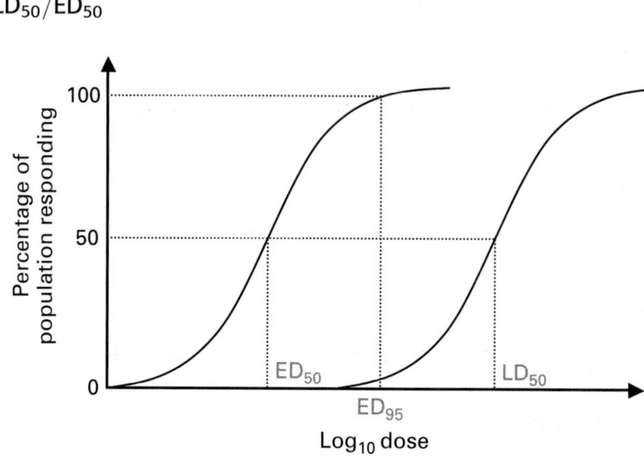

Both curves are sigmoid as before, The curve on the left represents a normal dosing regimen aiming to achieve the desired effect. Label the ED_{50} on it as before. The curve to the right represents a higher dosing regimen at which fatalities begin to occur in the test population. The LD_{50} should be at its midpoint. The ED_{95} is also marked on this graph; this is the point at which 95% of the population will have shown the desired response to dosing. However, note that by this stage some fatalities have already started to occur and the curves overlap. You can draw the curves more widely separated if you wish to avoid this but it is useful to demonstrate that a dose that is safe for one individual in a population may cause serious side effects to another.

Agonism and antagonism

Agonist

A drug which binds to a specific receptor (affinity) and, once bound, is able to produce a response (intrinsic activity).

Antagonist

A drug that has significant affinity but no intrinsic activity.

Full agonist

A drug that produces a maximal response once bound to the receptor.

Partial agonist

A drug with significant affinity but submaximal intrinsic activity.

Partial agonist curves

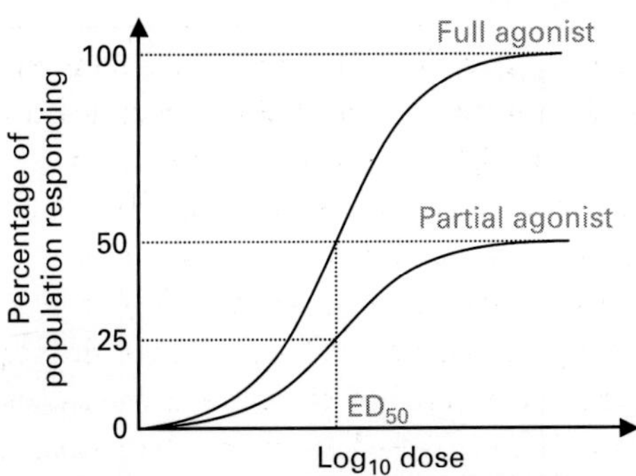

Draw a standard log-dose versus response curve as before and label it 'full agonist'. Next draw a second sigmoid curve that does not rise so far on the *y* axis. The inability to reach 100% population response automatically makes this representative of a partial agonist as it lacks efficacy. The next thing to consider is potency. The ED_{50} is taken as the point that lies half way between baseline and the maximum population response. For a full agonist, this is always half of 100%, but for a partial agonist it is half whatever the maximum is. In this instance, the maximum population response is 50% and so the ED_{50} is read at 25%. In this plot, both the agonist and partial agonist are equally potent as they share the same ED_{50}.

Partial agonist curve

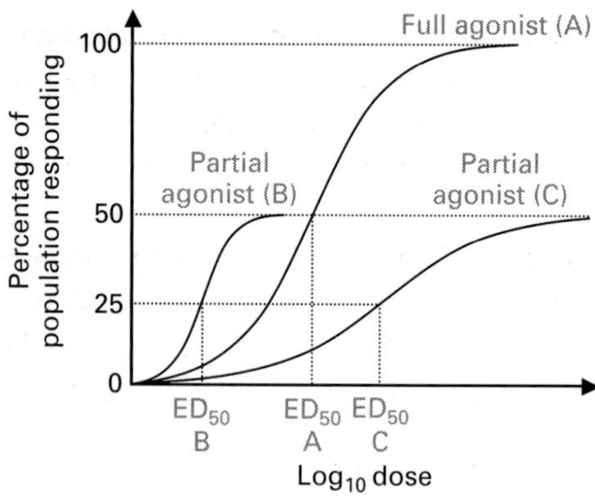

This graph enables you to demonstrate how the partial agonist curves change with changes in potency. Curve A is the standard sigmoid agonist curve. Curve B is plotted so that its ED_{50} is reduced compared with that of A. Drug B is, therefore, more potent than drug A but less efficacious. Curve C demonstrates an ED_{50} that is higher than that of curve A, and so drug C is less potent than drug A and less efficacious.

Alternative partial agonist curve

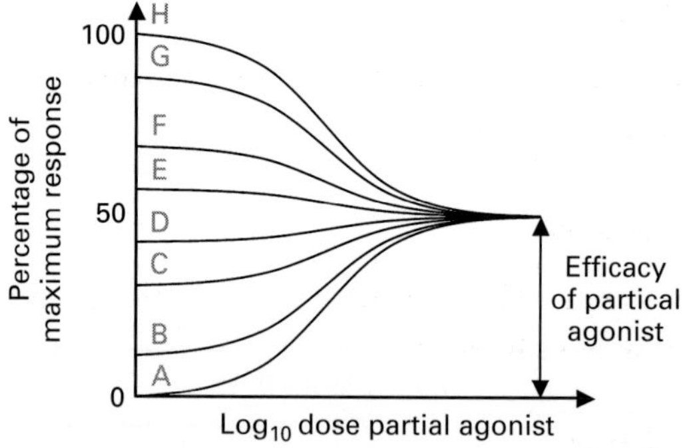

Partial agonists can also behave as antagonists, as demonstrated by this graph. The graph is constructed by starting with a number of different concentrations (A–H) of full agonist to which a partial agonist is successively added. The curves are best explained by describing the lines at the two extremes, 'A' and 'H'. Lines B–G demonstrate intermediate effects.

Line H This line shows a high baseline full agonist concentration and so begins with 100% maximal response. As an increasing dose of partial agonist is added, it displaces the full agonist from the receptors until eventually they are only able to generate the maximal response of the partial agonist (in this case 50%). The partial agonist has, therefore, behaved as an antagonist by preventing the maximal response that would have been seen with a full agonist alone.

Line A This line shows the opposite effect where there is no initial full agonist present and hence no initial response. As more partial agonist is added, the response rises to the maximum possible (50%) and so in this instance the partial agonist has behaved as an agonist by increasing the response seen.

Competitive antagonist

A compound that competes with endogenous agonists for the same binding site; it may be reversible or irreversible.

Non-competitive antagonist

A compound that binds at a different site to the natural receptor and produces a conformational distortion that prevents receptor activation.

Reversible antagonist

A compound whose inhibitory effects may be overcome by increasing the concentration of an agonist.

Irreversible antagonist

A compound whose inhibitory effects cannot be overcome by increasing the concentration of an agonist.

Allosteric modulator

An allosteric modulator binds at a site different from the natural receptor and alters the affinity of the receptor for the ligand, thus increasing or decreasing the effect of the natural agonist.

Reversible competitive antagonist curves

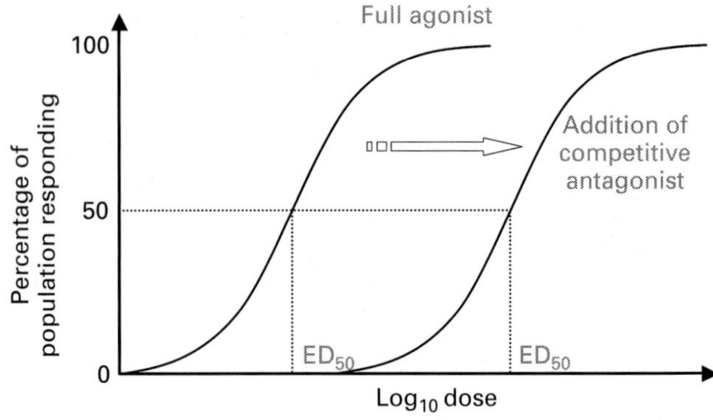

Draw the standard sigmoid curve and label it as a full agonist. Draw a second identical curve displaced to the right. This represents the new [DR] curve for an agonist in the presence of a competitive antagonist. The antagonist has blocked receptor sites; consequently, more agonist must be added to displace antagonist and achieve the same response. Demonstrate this by marking the ED_{50} on the graph and showing that potency of the agonist decreases in the presence of a competitive antagonist.

Irreversible competitive antagonist curves

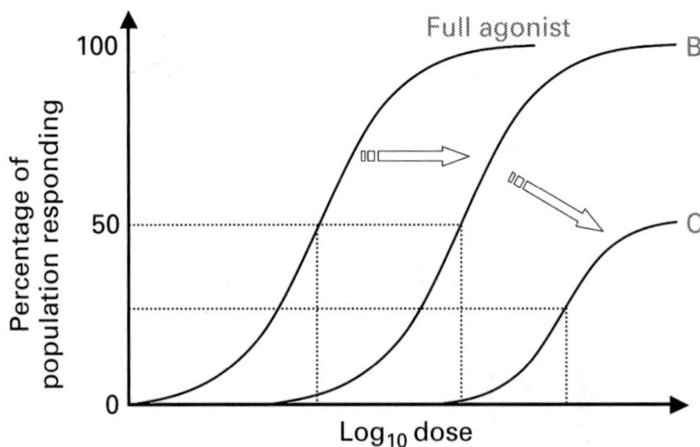

The standard curve is displaced to the right initially as some receptor sites are blocked by the antagonist. Given enough agonist, maximum response is still possible (line B) at the expense of reduced potency. With higher levels of antagonist present (line C), the potency and efficacy are both reduced as too many receptor sites are blocked by the antagonist to enable maximum response. With the addition of enough antagonist, no response will be seen.

Non-competitive antagonist curve

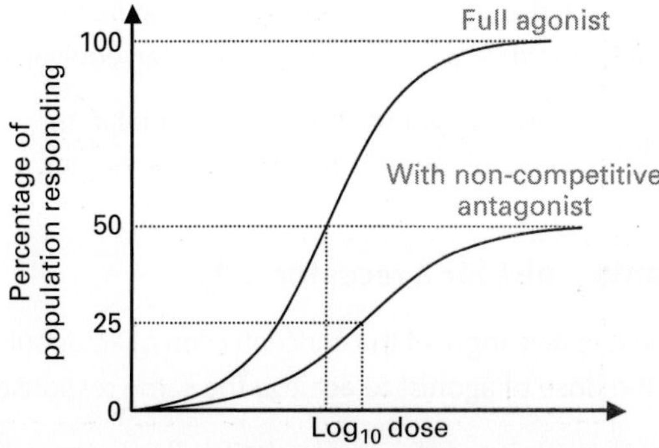

Because a non-competitive antagonist alters the shape of the receptor, the agonist cannot bind at all. The usual sigmoid curve is displaced down and to the right in a similar manner to the graph of agonist versus partial agonist drawn above. Increasing the dose of agonist does not improve response as receptor sites are no longer available for binding.

Inverse agonist

A compound that, when bound, produces an effect opposite to the endogenous agonist.

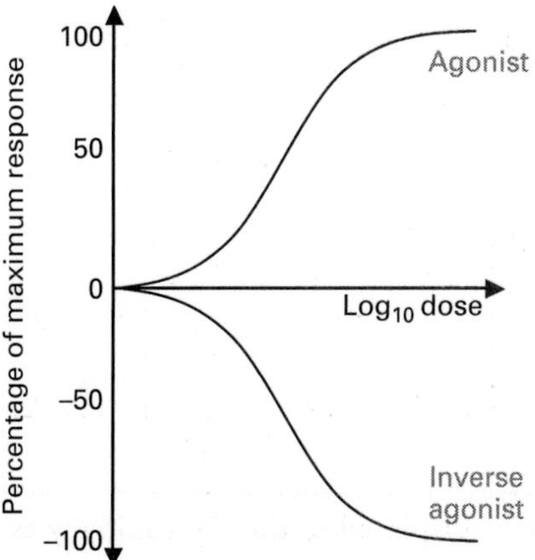

This plot is more theoretical than most. Draw the *y* axis so that it enables positive and 'negative' response. The upper curve is a standard sigmoid full agonist curve. The lower curve represents the action of the inverse agonist and should be plotted as an inverted curve. This is different from the curve of a pure antagonist, which would simply produce no effect rather than the opposite effect to a full agonist.

Dose ratio

The factor by which the agonist concentration must be increased when in the presence of a competitive antagonist to produce an equivalent response:

$$\text{Dose ratio} = \frac{\text{Dose of agonist in presence of inhibitor}}{\text{Dose of agonist in absence of inhibitor}}$$

Affinity of an antagonist for a receptor: pA_2

The pA_2 is the negative $\log_{10}$ of the concentration of antagonist that requires a doubling of the dose of agonist to achieve the same response.

It is a measure of the affinity of the antagonist for the receptor (the equilibrium dissociation constant). It is used to compare the potency of antagonists in a similar manner to the use of the ED_{50} to compare the potency of agonists.

Hysteresis

Hysteresis is defined on p. 14 but occurs in pharmacology as well as during physical measurement. The phenomenon occurs because the concentration of a drug at the intended site of action (the 'effector site' or 'biophase') often differs from the plasma concentration at any given time. The reasons for this time lag include the degree of ionization of the drug, its lipid solubility, prevailing concentration gradients and many other factors. All these alter the length of time it actually takes a drug to reach its intended site of action.

If a drug was to be administered orally, the following graph may be obtained.

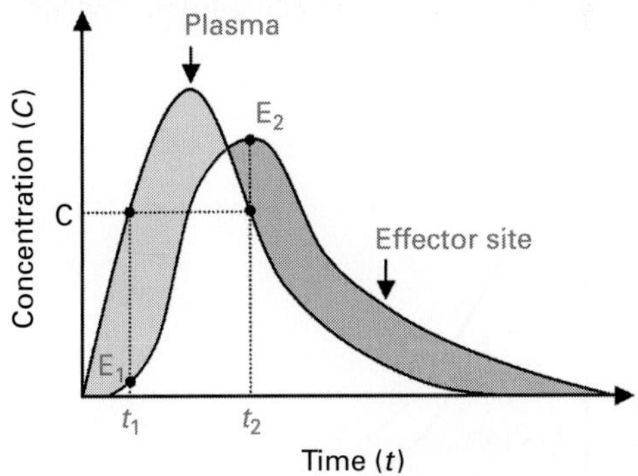

Plasma After drawing and labelling the axes, plot the concentration versus time curve for an orally administered drug. Label this curve 'plasma' to show how the concentration rises and falls with time following an oral dose.

Effector site Now draw a second, similar curve to the right of the first. This shows the concentration of the drug at its site of action. The degree of displacement to the right of the first curve is determined by the factors mentioned above.

Key points When both curves are drawn, mark a fixed concentration point on the y axis and label it C. Demonstrate that the plasma concentration curve crosses this value twice, at times t_1 and t_2. At time t_1 the concentration in the plasma is rising and at t_2 it is falling. The crucial point now that enables you to define hysteresis is to demonstrate that the effector site concentration is different at these two times depending on whether the plasma concentration is rising (giving concentration E_1) or falling (giving concentration E_2).

Bioavailability

Bioavailability is defined as the fraction of drug that reaches the circulation compared with the same dose given intravenously (i.v.) (%).

or

The ratio of the area under the stated concentration–time curve (AUC) divided by the area under the i.v. concentration–time curve.

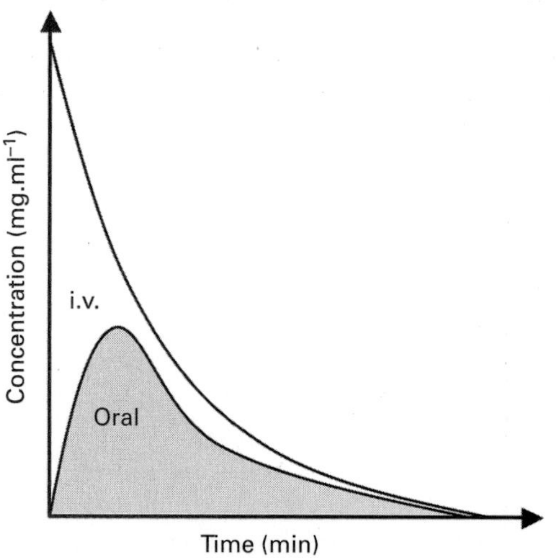

Intravenous After drawing and labelling the axes, plot an exponential decline curve to show how concentration changes with time following the i.v. administration of a drug. Note that the graph assumes a single compartment (see below). Although the concentration at time zero is not possible to measure, it is still conventional to plot the curve crossing the *y* axis. If you are asked how to calculate this initial concentration, it requires you to perform a semi-log transformation on the curve and to extrapolate the resultant straight line back to the *y* axis.

Oral Draw a second curve that shows the concentration of the same drug changing with time following its oral administration. The second curve does not have to be contained entirely within the i.v. curve although this is often the case in practice.

Extraction ratio

Fraction of total drug removed from the blood by an organ in each pass through that organ.

Volume of distribution

Volume of distribution

The theoretical volume into which a drug distributes following its administration (ml)

$$V_D = \frac{\text{Dose}}{C_0}$$

where V_D is the volume of distribution and C_0 is the concentration at time 0.

It is not possible to measure C_0 since mixing is not instantaneous; therefore, a semi-logarithmic plot is drawn and extrapolated back to the *y* axis in order to calculate this concentration.

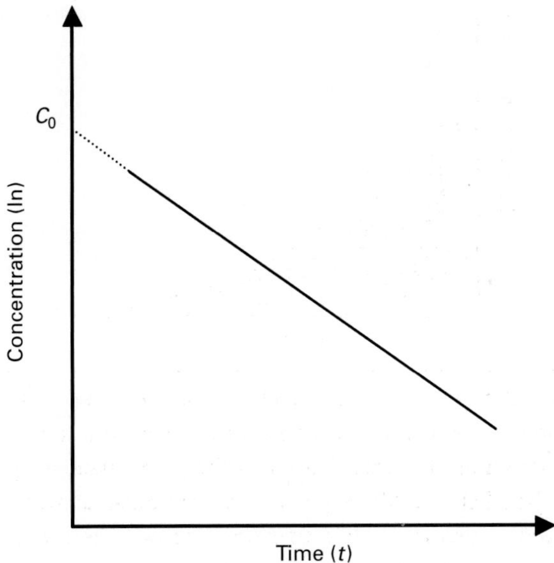

After drawing and labelling the axes as shown, plot a straight line (solid) which does not cross the *y* axis. This will be the curve which is found in the real world situation. To calculate C_0 the line must be extrapolated back (dotted) to the *y* axis and the concentration read at that point.

Using a simple one-compartment model, the loading dose and the infusion rate required to maintain a constant plasma concentration can be calculated as follows.

$$LD = V_D.C$$

where LD is the loading dose and C is the required plasma concentration.

and

$$R_{inf} = C.Cl$$

where R_{inf} is the infusion rate required and Cl is the clearance.

Clearance

Clearance

The volume of plasma from which a drug is removed per unit time ($ml.min^{-1}$).

It is important to remember that clearance refers to the amount of plasma concerned as opposed to the amount of a drug. Try to remember the units of $ml.min^{-1}$, which, in turn, should help you to remember the definition:

$$Cl = \frac{Dose}{AUC}$$

where AUC is the area under concentration–time curve

or

$$Cl = Q.ER$$

where Q is the flow rate and ER is the extraction ratio.

Clearance gives a value for the amount of plasma cleared of a drug. The mechanism of this clearance can involve elimination, excretion or both.

Elimination

Removal of drug from the plasma. This may be via distribution, metabolism or excretion.

$$R_{elim} = \text{Concentration} \times \text{Clearance}$$

or

$$R_{elim} = V_D \times K_{elim}$$

R_{elim} is the rate of elimination and K_{elim} is the rate constant of elimination.

First-order elimination

A situation where the rate of drug elimination at any time depends upon the concentration of the drug present at that time.

This is an exponential process and a constant *proportion* of drug is eliminated in a given time.

Zero-order elimination

A situation where the rate of drug elimination is independent of the concentration of drug and is, therefore, constant.

This time a constant *amount* of drug is eliminated in a given time rather than a constant proportion. First-order elimination may become zero order when the elimination system (often a metabolic pathway) is saturated.

Excretion

The removal of drug from the body.

Compartmental models

The concept of compartmental modelling allows predictions of drug behaviour to be made from mathematical models of the body that are more accurate than the assumption of the body being a simple container.

Compartment

> One or more components of a mathematical model that aim to replicate the drug-handling characteristics of a proportion of the body.

Models may contain any number of compartments but single-compartment models are generally inaccurate for studying pharmacokinetics. A three-compartment model allows fairly accurate modelling with only limited complexity.

Catenary

> A form of multicompartmental modelling in which all compartments are linked in a linear chain with each compartment connecting only to its immediate neighbour.

Mamillary

> A form of multicompartmental modelling in which there is a central compartment to which a stated number of peripheral compartments are connected.

Mamillary models are the most commonly used and are described below.

One-compartment model

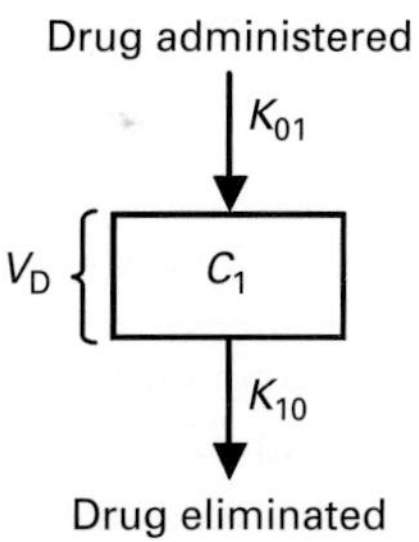

> The terminology for the so-called 'central' compartment is C_1. There are various rate constants that should be included in the diagram: K_{01} is the rate constant for a drug moving from the outside of the body (compartment 0) to the central compartment (compartment 1); K_{10} is the rate constant of elimination from C_1 to C_0. Single-compartment models do not occur physiologically.

Two-compartment model

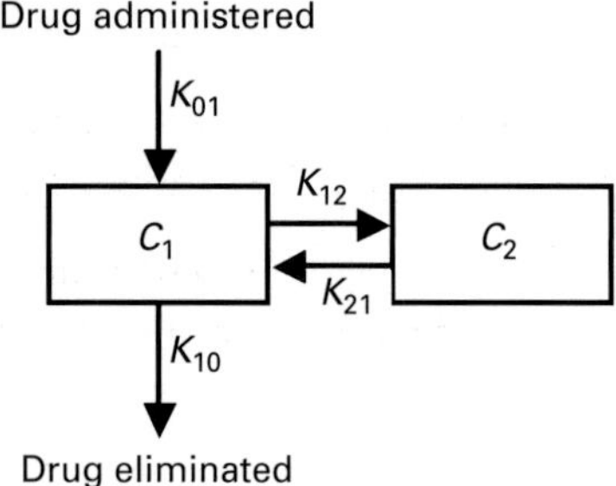

A second (peripheral) compartment can now be added, which may mathematically represent the less vascular tissues of the body. All the rate constants that were in the previous model still apply but in addition you must indicate that there are additional constants relating to this new compartment. The terminology is the same; K_{12} represents drug distribution from C_1 to C_2 and K_{21} represents drug redistribution back into C_1. Demonstrate in your diagram that elimination occurs only from C_1 no matter how many other compartments are present.

A semi-log plot of drug concentration versus time will no longer be linear as the drug has two possible paths to move along, each with their own associated rate constants.

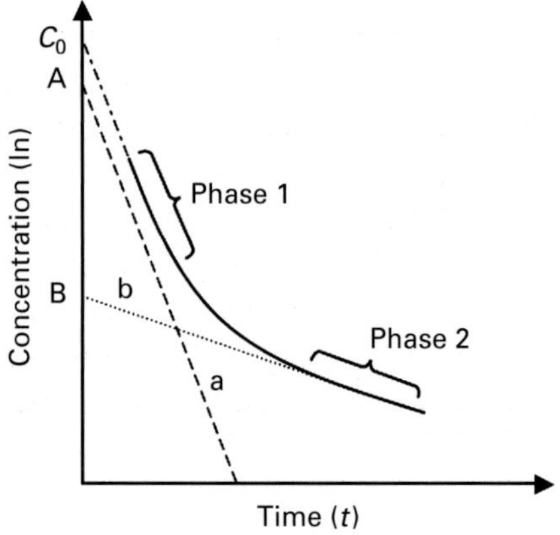

To show the concentration time curve for two compartments, first draw and label the axes as on p. 106. Instead of being linear, a bi-exponential curve should be drawn. Phase 1 equates to distribution of drug from C_1 to C_2 whereas phase 2 represents drug elimination from C_1. A tangent (b) to phase 2 intercepts the y axis at B. Subtracting line b from the initial curve gives line a, which intercepts the y axis at A and is a tangent to phase 1. The values of A and B sum to give C_0. Because the scale is logarithmic on the y axis, B is small in comparison with A and, therefore, C_0 and A are close.

Formula for two-compartment model

$$C_t = A.e^{-\alpha t} + B.e^{-\beta t}$$

where C_t is the concentration at time t, A is the y intercept of line a, α is the slope of line a, B is the y intercept of line b and β is the slope of line b.

The value of C_t can, therefore, be found simply by adding the values of exponential declines a and b at any given time. The terms α and β are the rate constants for these processes.

Three-compartment model

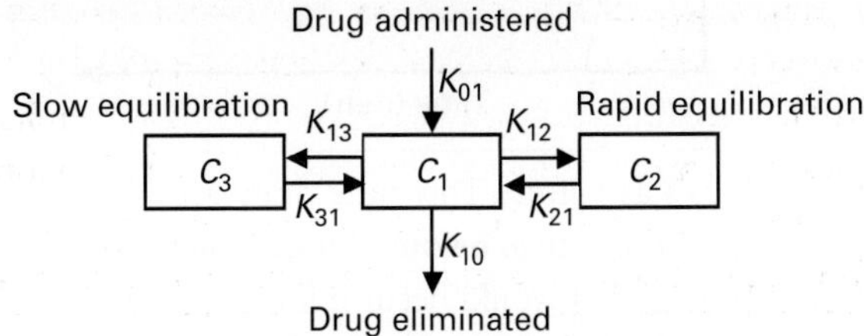

A third compartment can now be added that mathematically represents the least vascular tissues of the body. All the rate constants that were in the previous model still apply but in addition you must indicate that there are additional constants relating to this new compartment. The terminology is the same. Demonstrate in your diagram that elimination occurs only from C_1 no matter how many other compartments are present. Most anaesthetic drugs are accurately modelled in this way. Remember that the compartments are not representing precise physiological regions of the body. Instead they are designed to model areas of the body that share similar properties in terms of rates of equilibration with the central compartment. Your diagram should show, however, that one of the peripheral compartments models slowly equilibrating tissues while the other models tissues that are equilibrating more rapidly.

Concentration versus time

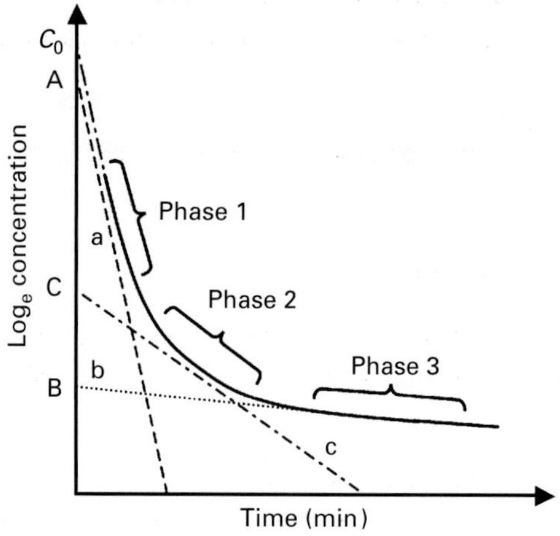

Draw and label the axes as before. This time draw a tri-exponential decline. Draw a tangent to phase 3 (line b) as before giving a y intercept at B. Next draw a tangent to phase 2 (line c) that would occur if line b were subtracted from the original tri-exponential decline. Show that this line intercepts the y axis at C. Finally draw a tangent to phase 1 (line a), which would occur if lines b and c were subtracted from the original tri-exponential decline. Show that this intercepts the y axis at A. As before, $A + B + C$ should equal C_0. Line a represents distribution to rapidly equilibrating tissues and line c represents distribution to slowly equilibrating tissues. Line b always represents elimination from the body.

Formula for three-compartment model

$$C_t = A.e^{-\alpha t} + B.e^{-\beta t} + C.e^{-\gamma t}$$

where C is the y intercept of line c and γ is the slope of line c.

The equation is compiled in the same way as that for a two-compartment model: $B.e^{-\beta t}$ continues to represent the terminal elimination phase and the term $C.e^{-\gamma t}$ is added to represent slowly equilibrating compartments.

Three-compartment models show how drug first enters a central (first) compartment, is then distributed rapidly to a second and slowly to a third whilst being eliminated only from the first. Distribution to, and redistribution from, the peripheral compartments occurs continuously according to prevailing concentration gradients. These peripheral compartments may act as reservoirs keeping the central compartment full even as elimination is occurring from it. The ratio of the rate constants to and from the central compartment will, therefore, affect the length of time taken to eliminate a drug fully.

Context-sensitive half time

The use of compartmental models leads onto the subject of context-sensitive half time (CSHT).

Context-sensitive half time

The time taken for the plasma concentration of a drug to fall by half after the cessation of an infusion designed to maintain a steady plasma concentration (time).

Although there is not a recognized definition for the term 'context', it is used to identify the fact that the half time will usually alter in the setting of varying *durations* of drug infusion.

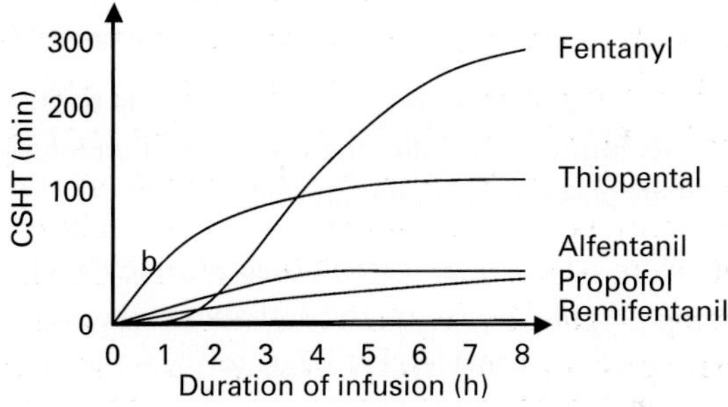

Draw and label the axes as shown. In terms of accuracy, it is often easiest to draw in the curves from the drugs with the shortest CSHT first before plotting the others.

Remifentanil This is the exceptional drug in anaesthetic practice in that it is context *insensitive*. Draw a straight line starting from the origin and becoming near horizontal after the CSHT reaches 5 min. This demonstrates that the half time is not dependent on the length of infusion as clearance by plasma esterases is so rapid.

Propofol Starting at the origin, draw a smooth curve rising steadily towards a CSHT of around 40 min after 8 h of infusion. Propofol is not context insensitive as its CSHT continues to rise; however it remains short even after prolonged infusions.

Alfentanil The curve rises from the origin until reaching a CSHT of 50 min at around 2 h of infusion. Thereafter the curve becomes horizontal. This demonstrates that alfentanil is also context insensitive for infusion durations of 2 h or longer.

Thiopental The curve begins at the origin but rises more steeply than the others so that the CSHT is 50 min after only 30 min infusion duration. The curve should be drawn like a slightly slurred build-up exponential reaching a CSHT of 150 min after 8 h of infusion. As the CSHT continues to rise, thiopental does not become context insensitive.

Fentanyl The most complex curve begins at the origin and is sigmoid in shape. It should cross the alfentanil line at 2 h duration and rise to a CSHT of 250 min after 6 h of infusion. Again, as the CSHT continues to rise, fentanyl does not become context insensitive.

It is important to realize that the CSHT does not predict the time to patient awakening but simply the time until the plasma concentration of a drug has fallen by half. The patient may need the plasma concentration to fall by 75% in order to awaken, and the time taken for this or any other percentage fall to occur is known as a decrement time.

Decrement time

The time taken for the plasma concentration of a drug to fall to the specified percentage of its former value after the cessation of an infusion designed to maintain a steady plasma concentration (time).

The CSHT is, therefore, a form of decrement time when the 'specified percentage' is 50%. When using propofol infusions, the decrement time is commonly quoted as the time taken to reach a plasma level of 1.2 $\mu g.ml^{-1}$, as this is the level at which wake up is thought likely to occur in the absence of any other sedative agents.

Lung volumes

Most lung volumes can be measured with a spirometer except total lung capacity (TLC), functional residual capacity (FRC) and residual volume (RV). The FRC can be measured by helium dilution or body plethysmography.

Tidal volume (TV)

The volume of gas which is inhaled or exhaled during the course of a normal resting breath. Also represented by the symbol V_T (ml).

Residual volume (RV)

The volume of gas that remains in the lungs after a maximal forced expiration (ml).

Inspiratory reserve volume (IRV)

The volume of gas that can be further inhaled after the end of a normal tidal inhalation (ml).

Expiratory reserve volume (ERV)

The volume of gas that can be further exhaled after the end of a normal tidal exhalation (ml).

Capacity

The sum of one of more lung volumes.

Vital capacity (VC)

The volume of gas inhaled when a maximal expiration is followed immediately by a maximal inspiration. The sum of the ERV, IRV and TV (ml).

Functional residual capacity (FRC)

The volume of gas that remains in the lungs after a normal tidal expiration. It is the sum of the ERV and the RV (ml).

You may be asked for the definitions above, and to explain them clearly it is often useful to refer to a diagram. You will be expected to be familiar with a diagram of normal respiratory volumes against time, and to be able to explain its main components.

Lung volumes

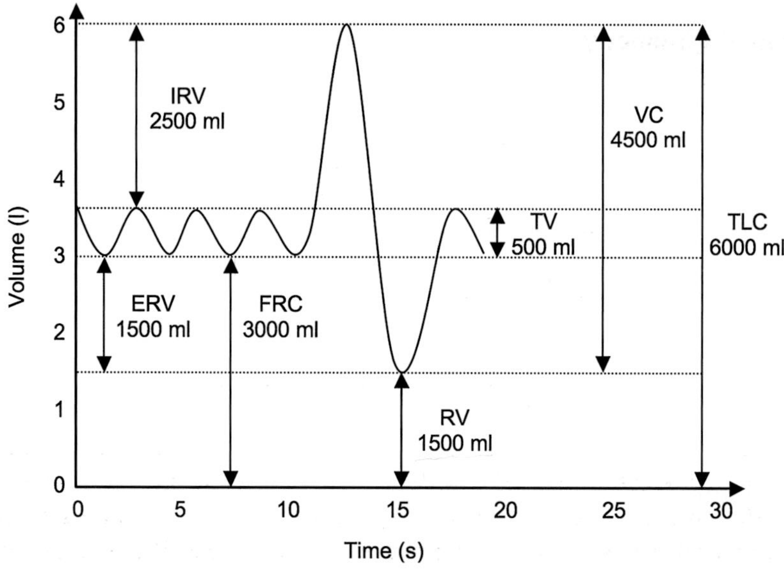

As the FRC is around 3000 ml, the TV should be drawn as an undulating line with its baseline at 3000 ml rising to 3500 ml on inspiration. Consider, and be prepared to explain, how the curve would shift in pathological situations. For example, in asthmatics the FRC may increase while the IRV decreases as a consequence of gas trapping.

Closing volume

> The volume of gas remaining in the lung when the small airways start to close (ml).

It is calculated by measuring the nitrogen concentration in expired gas after a single breath of 100% oxygen. The nitrogen wash-out test is the same method used to measure anatomical dead space. Closing volume increases with age and reaches the standing FRC at 70 years and the supine FRC at 40 years.

Spirometry

Simple spirometry using a Vitalograph or similar produces a well-defined curve that can aid in the interpretation of various lung diseases.

Normal spirometry

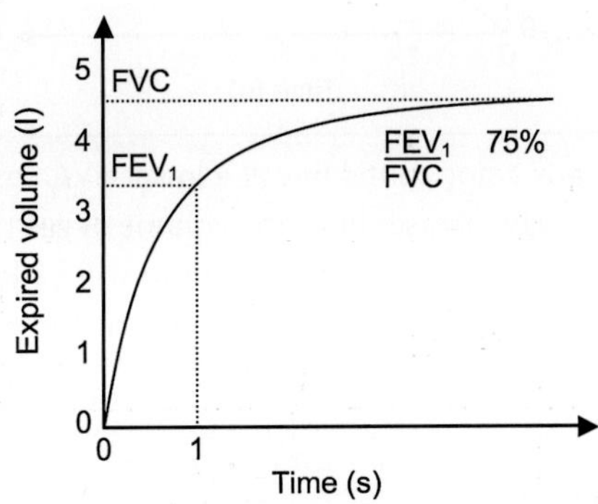

Draw and label the axes as shown. Next draw a horizontal line at the level of the forced vital capacity (FVC; 4500 ml) to act as a target point for where the curve must end. Normal physiology allows for 75% of the FVC to be forcibly expired in 1 s (FEV_1) . The normal FEV_1 should, therefore, be 3375 ml. Mark this volume at a time of 1 s. Construct the curve by drawing a smooth arc passing through the FEV_1 point and coming into alignment with the FVC line at the other end.

Obstructive pattern

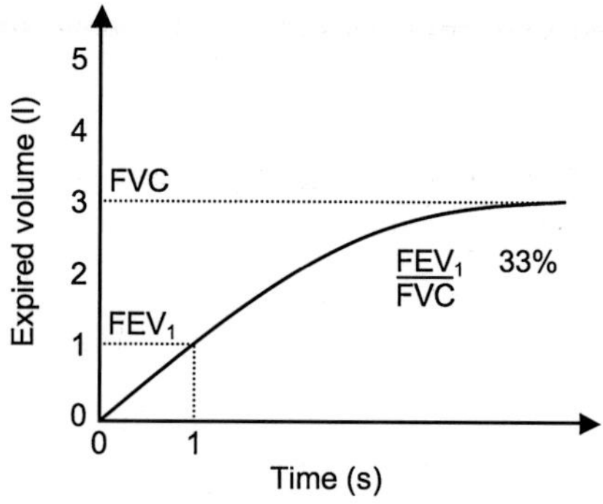

On the same axes, draw a horizontal line at a lower FVC to act as a target end point. Obstructive airway diseases limit the volume of gas that can be forcibly expired in 1 s and, therefore, the FEV_1/FVC ratio will be lower. In the graph above, the ratio is 33% giving a FEV_1 of 1000 ml for a FVC of 3000 ml. Construct the curve in the same way as before.

Restrictive pattern

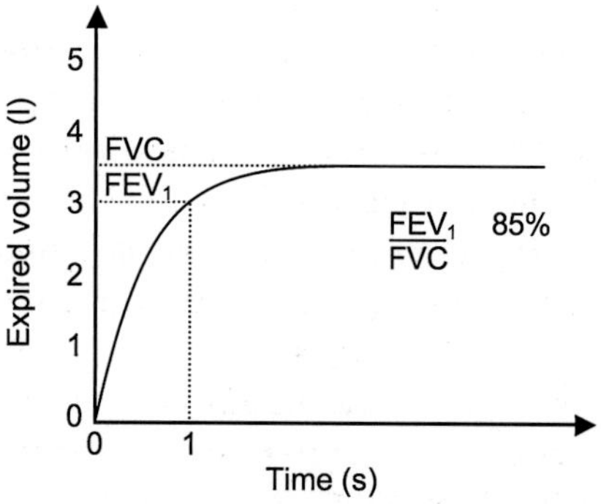

On the same axes, draw a horizontal line at a lower FVC than normal to act as a target end point. Restrictive lung disease curtails the FVC but generally does not affect early expiration. For this reason, the FEV_1/FVC ratio is normal or high. In the graph above, the ratio is 85%, giving a FEV_1 of 3000 ml for a FVC of 3500 ml. Construct the curve in the same way as before.

Flow–volume loops

You should be able to draw the following loops as examples of various respiratory system pathologies.

Normal loop

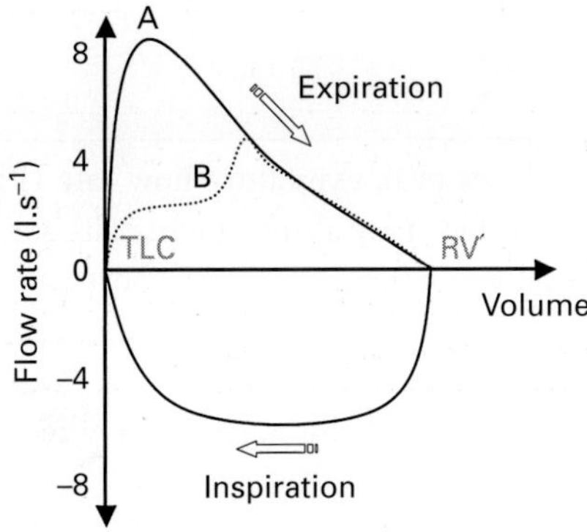

Draw and label the axes as shown; the *x* axis need not display numerical values but a note should be made of the TLC and RV. Note that the highest volume (TLC) is on the left of the *x* axis. The units on the *y* axis are litres per second as opposed to litres per minute. Positive deflection occurs during expiration and negative deflection during inspiration. The patient takes a VC breath before starting the test with a forced expiration. The loop is drawn in a clockwise direction starting from TLC. The normal loop (A) rises rapidly to a flow rate of 8–10 l.s^{-1} at the start of forced expiration. The flow rate then decreases steadily as expiration continues in a left to right direction so that a relatively straight curve is produced with a slight concavity at its centre. An important point to demonstrate is the phenomenon of dynamic compression of the airways. The curve traced by the normal loop represents the maximum possible flow rate at each lung volume. Even if patients 'holds back' their maximal effort by expiring slowly at first (B), they will be unable to cross this maximal flow line. This is because the airways are compressed by a rise in intrathoracic pressure, thus limiting flow. The more effort that is put into expiration, the more these airways are compressed and so total flow remains the same. The inspiratory limb has a much squarer shape to it and a maximum flow of 4–6 l.s^{-1} is usually achieved. Inspiration occurs from RV to TLC in a right to left direction as shown.

Obstructive disease

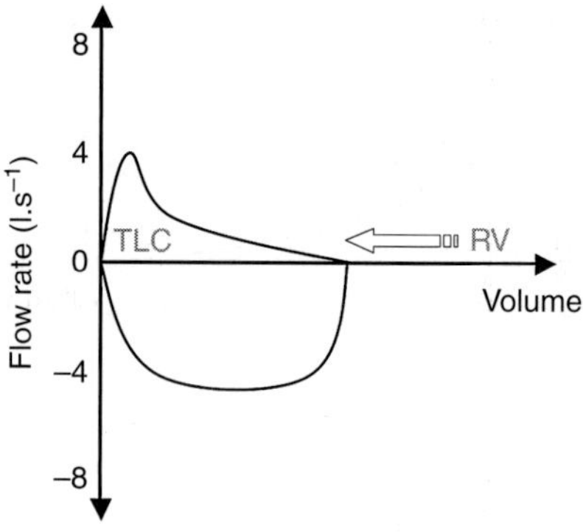

Obstructive disease reduces peak expiratory flow rate (PEFR) and increases RV via gas trapping. The TLC may also be higher although this is difficult to demonstrate without values on the *x* axis. The important point to demonstrate is reduced flow rates during all of expiration, with increased concavity of the expiratory limb owing to airway obstruction. The inspiratory limb is less affected and can be drawn as for the normal curve but with slightly lower flow rates.

Restrictive disease

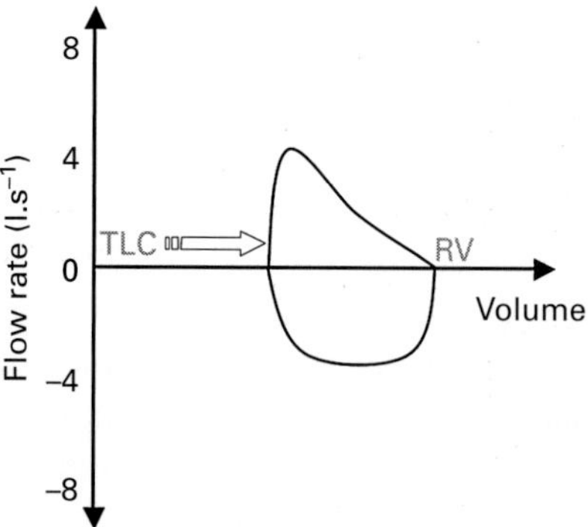

In contrast to obstructive disease, restrictive disease markedly reduces TLC while preserving RV. The PEFR is generally reduced. Demonstrate these points by drawing a curve that is similar in shape to the normal curve but in which the flow rates are reduced. In addition, the left-hand side of the curve is shifted to the right, demonstrating a fall in TLC.

Variable intrathoracic obstruction

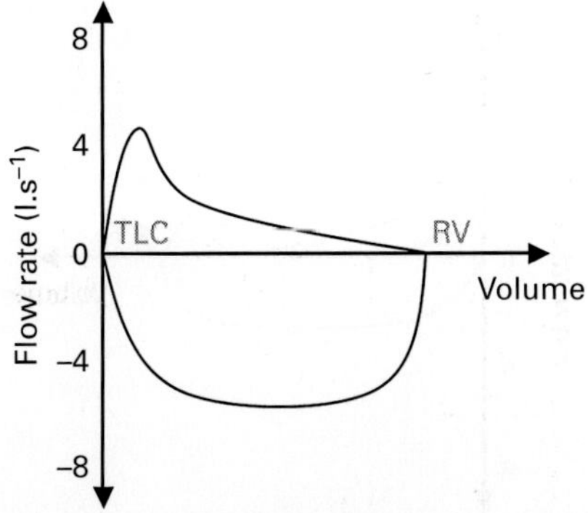

An intrathoracic obstruction is more likely to allow gas flow during inspiration as the negative intrathoracic pressure generated helps to pull the airways open. As such, the inspiratory limb of the curve may be near normal. In contrast, the positive pressure generated during forced expiration serves only to exacerbate the obstruction, and as such the expiratory limb appears similar to that seen in obstructive disease. Both TLC and RV are generally unaffected.

Variable extrathoracic obstruction

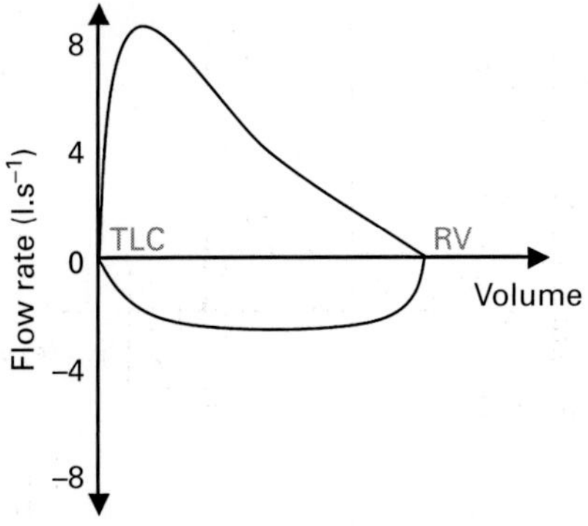

An extrathoracic obstruction is more likely to allow gas flow during expiration as the positive pressure generated during this phase acts to force the airway open. As such, the expiratory limb may be near normal. In contrast, the negative pressure generated in the airway during inspiration serves to collapse the airway further and the inspiratory limb will show markedly reduced flow rates at all volumes while retaining its square shape. Both TLC and RV are generally unaffected.

Fixed large airway obstruction

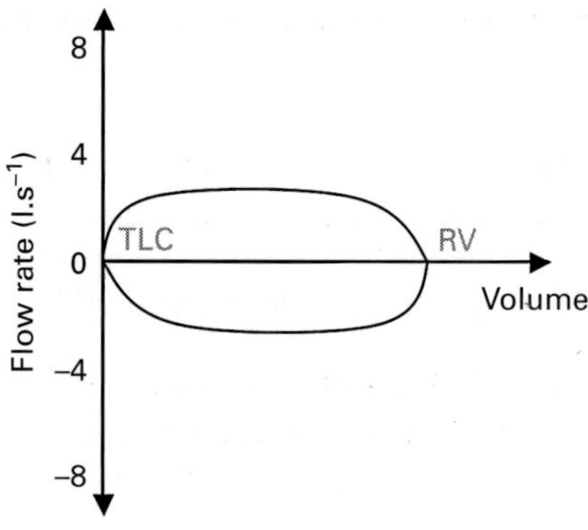

This curve is seen where a large airway has a fixed orifice through which gas is able to flow, such as may be seen in patients with tracheal stenosis. The peak inspiratory and expiratory flow rates are, therefore, dependent on the diameter of the orifice rather than effort. The curves should be drawn almost symmetrical as above, with both limbs demonstrating markedly reduced flow. The TLC and RV are generally unaffected.

The alveolar gas equation

The alveolar gas equation is used to estimate the P_{AO_2} of a 'perfect' alveolus with varying fractions of inspired oxygen and it states that

$$P_{AO_2} = [F_{IO_2} \times (P_{ATM} - P_{H_2O})] - (P_{ACO_2}/R)$$

where P_{AO_2} is the alveolar O_2 partial pressure, P_{ACO_2} is the alveolar CO_2 partial pressure, P_{ATM} is the atmospheric pressure, F_{IO_2} is the fraction of inspired air, P_{H_2O} is the standard vapour pressure (SVP) of water at 37 °C and R is the respiratory quotient.

Note that the SVP of water in the airways is subtracted from the atmospheric pressure before multiplying by the F_{IO_2}. This is because the fractional concentration of O_2 only applies to the portion of inhaled mixture that is dry gas.

The P_{ACO_2} is assumed to be in equilibrium with arterial CO_2 tension (P_{aCO_2}) and this number will either be given or will be assumed to be within the normal range.

The value of R varies according to which energy substrates make up the predominant part of the diet. With a normal diet, it is assumed to have a value of 0.8; pure carbohydrate metabolism gives a value of 1.0.

Therefore, under normal conditions:

$$\begin{aligned} P_{AO_2} &= [0.21 \times (101.3 - 6.3)] - (5.3/0.8) \\ &= (0.21 \times 95) - 6.6 \\ &= 19.95 - 6.6 \\ &= 13.35 \text{ kPa} \end{aligned}$$

Note that there is no difference between the ideal alveolar value and the normal arterial P_{aO_2} of 13.3 kPa. In practice a difference of up to 2 kPa is allowable owing to ventilation–perfusion ($\dot{V}/\dot{Q}$) mismatch and shunt.

The shunt equation

The purpose of the shunt equation is to give a *ratio* of shunt blood flow to total blood flow. The normal ratio is 0.3. Under abnormal conditions, the ratio will tend to increase and so markedly reduce the Pa_{O_2}.

Shunt

Those areas of the lung that are perfused but not ventilated:

$$\frac{\dot{Q}_S}{\dot{Q}_T} = \frac{(Cc'_{O_2} - Ca_{O_2})}{(Cc'_{O_2} - C\bar{v}_{O_2})}$$

where $\dot{Q}_T$ is total blood flow, $\dot{Q}_S$ is shunted blood flow, Cc'_{O_2} is end-capillary blood content, $C\bar{v}_{O_2}$ is shunt blood O_2 content and Ca_{O_2} is arterial blood O_2 content.

Principle of the shunt equation

Start with the theoretical lungs shown above and remember that blood entering the systemic circulation has a component that is shunted past the pulmonary circulation ($\dot{Q}_S$) and another component that passes through it ($\dot{Q}_T - \dot{Q}_S$).

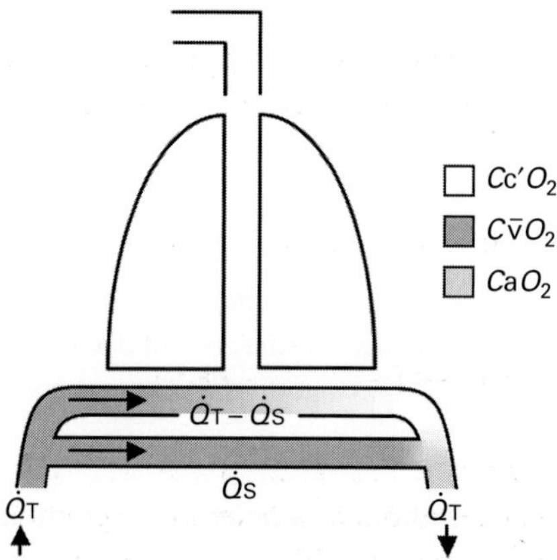

Now consider the blood flow generated in a single beat. The O_2 delivered in this volume of blood is equal to ($\dot{Q}_T.Ca_{O_2}$). This must be made up of shunted blood ($\dot{Q}_S.C\bar{v}_{O_2}$) and capillary blood ($[\dot{Q}_T - \dot{Q}_S].Cc'_{O_2}$).

$$\dot{Q}_T.Ca_{O_2} = (\dot{Q}_S.C\bar{v}_{O_2}) + [(\dot{Q}_T - \dot{Q}_S).Cc'_{O_2}]$$

Derivation

$$\dot{Q}_T.Ca_{O_2} = (\dot{Q}_S.C\bar{v}_{O_2}) + [(\dot{Q}_T - \dot{Q}_S).Cc'_{O_2}]$$

Rearrange the brackets to give

$$\dot{Q}_T.Ca_{O_2} = (\dot{Q}_S.C\bar{v}_{O_2}) + (\dot{Q}_T.Cc'_{O_2}) - (\dot{Q}_S.Cc'_{O_2})$$

$\dot{Q}_S$ needs to be moved to the left, aiming for $\dot{Q}_S/\dot{Q}_T$ in the final equation.

$$(\dot{Q}_T.Ca_{O_2}) + (\dot{Q}_S.Cc'_{O_2}) = (\dot{Q}_S.C\bar{v}_{O_2}) + (\dot{Q}_T.Cc'_{O_2})$$

then

$$(\dot{Q}_S.Cc'_{O_2}) = (\dot{Q}_S.C\bar{v}_{O_2}) + (\dot{Q}_T.Cc'_{O_2}) - (\dot{Q}_T.Ca_{O_2})$$

then

$$(\dot{Q}_S.Cc'_{O_2}) - (\dot{Q}_S.C\bar{v}_{O_2}) = (\dot{Q}_T.Cc'_{O_2}) - (\dot{Q}_T.Ca_{O_2})$$

Then simplify the brackets

$$\dot{Q}_S(Cc'_{O_2} - C\bar{v}_{O_2}) = \dot{Q}_T(Cc'_{O_2} - Ca_{O_2})$$

To get $\dot{Q}_S/\dot{Q}_T$ on the left, both sides must be divided by $\dot{Q}_T$. At the same time, the term $(Cc'_{O_2} - C\bar{v}_{O_2})$ can be moved from left to right by also dividing both sides by $(Cc'_{O_2} - C\bar{v}_{O_2})$.

$$\frac{\dot{Q}_S}{\dot{Q}_T} = \frac{(Cc'_{O_2} - Ca_{O_2})}{(Cc'_{O_2} - C\bar{v}_{O_2})}$$

The O_2 content of the mixed venous (shunt) and arterial blood can be calculated from the relevant samples by using the equations below, which are explained later in the section.

$$C\bar{v}_{O_2} = (1.34\,[\text{Hb}]\,\text{Sats}) + (0.0225\,.\,Pa_{O_2})$$

or

$$Ca_{O_2} = (1.34\,[\text{Hb}]\,\text{Sats}) + (0.0225\,.\,Pa_{O_2})$$

The value for Cc'_{O_2} cannot be calculated in this way very easily as a sample is technically difficult to take without a catheter in the pulmonary vein. It is, therefore, assumed to be in equilibrium with the P_{AO_2}, which, in turn, is given by the alveolar gas equation.

Pulmonary vascular resistance

Pulmonary vascular resistance (PVR) is given by:

$$PVR = \frac{(MPAP - LAP)}{CO} \times 80$$

where MPAP is mean pulmonary artery pressure, LAP is left atrial pressure and CO is cardiac output.

The units for PVR are dyne.s^{-1}.cm^{-5} and 80 is used as a conversion factor to account for the different units used within the equation

Factors affecting PVR

Increased by	Decreased by
Increased Pa_{CO_2}	Decreased Pa_{CO_2}
Decreased pH	Increased pH
Decreased Pa_{O_2}	Increased Pa_{O_2}
Adrenaline (epinephrine)	Isoprenaline
Noradrenaline (norepinephrine)	Acetylcholine
Thromboxane A_2	Prostacyclin (prostaglandin I_2)
Angiotensin II	Nitric oxide (NO)
Serotonin (5-hydroxytryptamine)	Increased peak airway pressure
Histamine	Increased pulmonary venous pressure
High or low lung volume	Volatile anaesthetic agents

Lung volume versus PVR graph

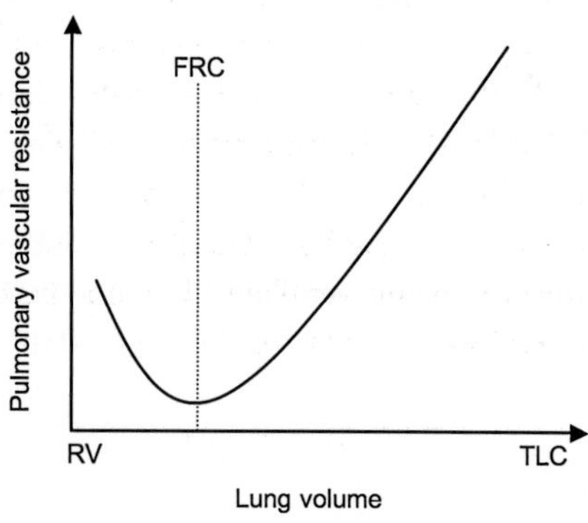

The point to demonstrate is that resistance is lowest around the FRC. The curve rises at low lung volumes as there is direct compression of the vessels. At high lung volumes, the vessels are overstretched, which alters the flow dynamics and increases resistance further. The curve will be moved up or down by those other factors (above) which increase or decrease PVR.

Ventilation/perfusion mismatch

The $\dot{V}/\dot{Q}$ term describes the imbalance between ventilation ($\dot{V}$) and perfusion ($\dot{Q}$) in different areas of the lung. Given that alveolar ventilation is $4.5\,l.min^{-1}$ and pulmonary arterial blood flow is $5.0\,l.min^{-1}$, the overall $\dot{V}/\dot{Q}$ ratio is 0.9. Both ventilation and perfusion increase from top to bottom of the lung, but perfusion by much more than ventilation.

Ventilation/perfusion graph

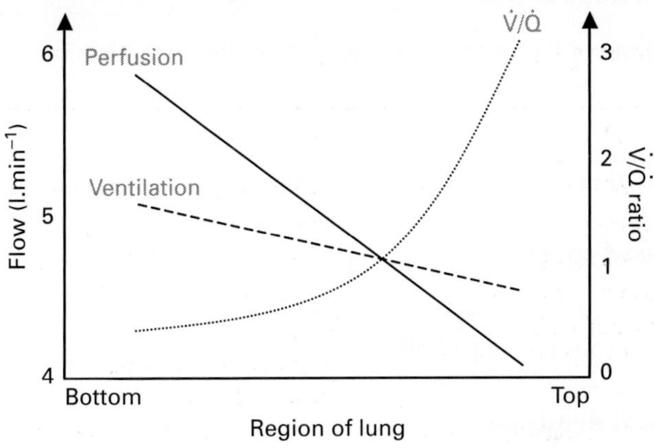

The graph can be drawn with either one or two *y* axes. The example above has two, flow and $\dot{V}/\dot{Q}$ ratio, and gives a slightly more complete picture. The *x* axis should be arranged from the bottom to the top regions of lung in a left to right direction as shown. Both ventilation and perfusion decrease linearly from bottom to top. Perfusion starts at a higher flow but decreases more rapidly than ventilation so that the lines cross approximately one third of the way down the lung. At this point the $\dot{V}/\dot{Q}$ ratio must be equal to 1. Using this point and a maximum $\dot{V}/\dot{Q}$ ratio of around 3, draw a smooth curve passing through both of these as it rises from left to right. The graph demonstrates that higher lung regions tend towards being ventilated but not perfused (dead space, $\dot{V}/\dot{Q} \approx \infty$) and lower regions tend towards being perfused but not ventilated (shunt, $\dot{V}/\dot{Q} \approx 0$).

Dead space

Dead space is an important concept in anaesthesia. As dead space increases, a smaller proportion of the inhaled gas mixture takes part in gas exchange.

Dead space

The volume of the airways in which no gas exchange occurs. It can be either anatomical or alveolar (ml).

Anatomical dead space

The volume of the conducting airways that does not contain any respiratory epithelium. This stretches from the nasal cavity to the generation 16 terminal bronchioles (ml).

The anatomical dead space can be measured by Fowler's method.

Alveolar dead space

The volume of those alveoli that are ventilated but not perfused, and so cannot take part in gas exchange (ml).

Physiological dead space

The sum of the anatomical and alveolar dead space (ml).

The physiological dead space can be calculated using the Bohr equation.

Fowler's method

Fowler's method principle

The patient takes a single vital capacity breath of O_2 and exhales through a N_2 analyser. Dead space gas, which is pure O_2, passes the analyser first, followed by a mixture of dead space and alveolar gas. When pure alveolar gas passes the analyser, a plateau is reached. At closing capacity, small airways begin to close, leading to preferential exhalation from the larger-diameter upper airways. These airways contain more N_2 as they are less well ventilated, so the initial concentration of N_2 within them was not diluted with O_2 during the O_2 breath.

Fowler's method graph

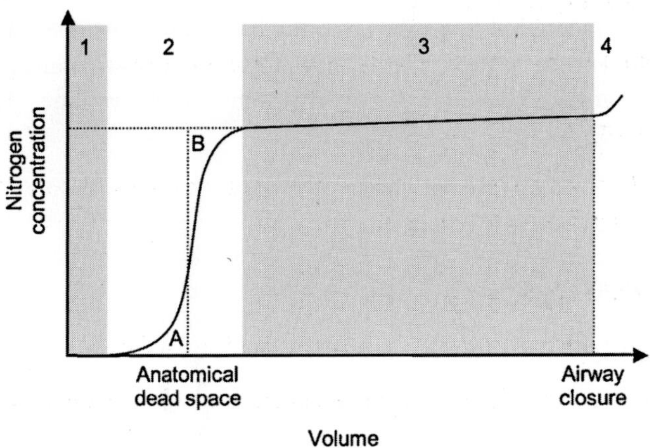

Phase 1 Pure dead space gas so no value on the *y* axis.

Phase 2 A mixture of dead space gas and alveolar gas. The curve rises steeply to a plateau. Demonstrate a vertical line that intercepts this curve such that area A equals area B. The anatomical dead space is taken as the volume expired at this point.

Phase 3 Plateau as alveolar gas with a steady N_2 content is exhaled. Note the curve is not completely horizontal during this stage.

Phase 4 Draw a final upstroke. This occurs at the closing volume. Note that the volume on the *x* axis at this point is not the value for the closing volume itself but rather the volume exhaled so far in the test. The closing volume represents the volume remaining within the lung at this point.

The Bohr equation

The purpose of the Bohr equation is to give a *ratio* of physiological dead space volume to tidal volume. Dead space volume is normally around 30% of tidal volume and so the normal ratio is quoted as 0.3. Under abnormal conditions, the ratio will tend to increase and so make ventilation inefficient.

The equation is:

$$V_D/V_T = (Pa_{CO_2} - P_{ECO_2})/Pa_{CO_2}$$

where V_D is the physiological dead space volume, V_T is the tidal volume, and P_{ECO_2} is the partial pressure of CO_2 in expired air.

Principle of the Bohr equation

Start with the theoretical lungs shown in the figure and remember that each V_T has a component that is dead space (V_D) and a remainder that must take part in gas exchange at the alveolus ($V_T - V_D$). This is the alveolar volume.

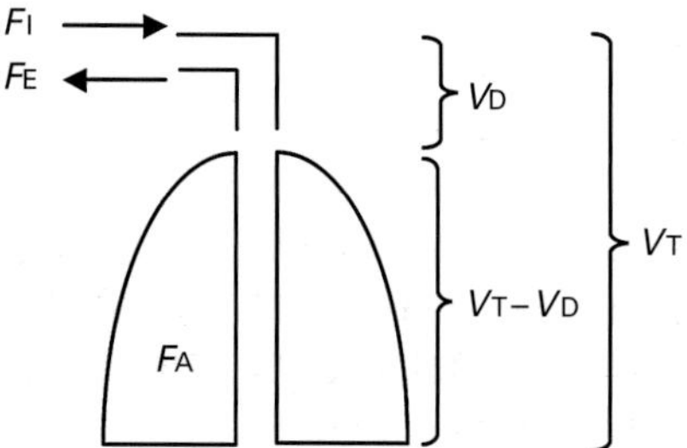

The fractional CO_2 concentrations are F_I for inhaled, F_E for exhaled and F_A for alveolar CO_2.

Now consider a single tidal exhalation. The CO_2 in this breath is equal to $F_E.V_T$. This must be made up of alveolar gas ($F_A\,[V_T - V_D]$) and dead space gas ($F_I.V_D$).

Derivation

$$F_E.V_T = (F_I.V_D) + (F_A[V_T - V_D])$$

But $F_I = 0$ so the term ($F_I.V_D$) can be ignored

$$F_E.V_T = F_A(V_T - V_D)$$

Rearrange the brackets to give

$$F_E.V_T = (F_A.V_T) - (F_A.V_D)$$

The term V_D needs to be moved to the left, aiming for V_D/V_T in the final equation. Start by adding ($F_A.V_D$) to both sides and subtracting ($F_E.V_T$) from both sides to give

$$(F_E.V_T) + (F_A.V_D) = F_A.V_T$$

or

$$F_A.V_D = (F_A.V_T) - (F_E.V_T)$$

Then simplify the brackets

$$F_A.V_D = V_T(F_A - F_E)$$

To get V_D/V_T on the left, both sides must be divided by V_T. At the same time, the term F_A can be moved from left to right by also dividing both sides by F_A

$$V_D/V_T = (F_A - F_E)/F_A$$

Since the concentration of a gas is proportional to its partial pressure (Dalton's law) F_A and F_E can be substituted for some more familiar units

$$F_A = P_{ACO_2}$$

$$F_E = P_{ECO_2}$$

Giving the Bohr equation as

$$V_D/V_T = (P_{ACO_2} - P_{ECO_2})/P_{ACO_2}$$

As arterial CO_2 tension is practically identical to alveolar CO_2 partial pressure, it can be used as a surrogate measurement. This is desirable as measuring arterial CO_2 tension involves only a simple blood gas analysis. The term P_{ACO_2}, therefore, becomes $Paco_2$ and so the equation is often written as

$$V_D/V_T = (Paco_2 - P_{ECO_2})/Paco_2$$

Some forms of the equation have the modifier $+[R]$ added to the end as a correction for high inspired CO_2.

Oxygen delivery and transport

Oxygen cascade

Oxygen flux is a term used to describe delivery of O_2 to the tissues. An understanding of how the $P\text{O}_2$ changes according to the location in the body is, therefore, useful when considering how the mitochondrial O_2 supply is achieved. It can be represented by the O_2 cascade.

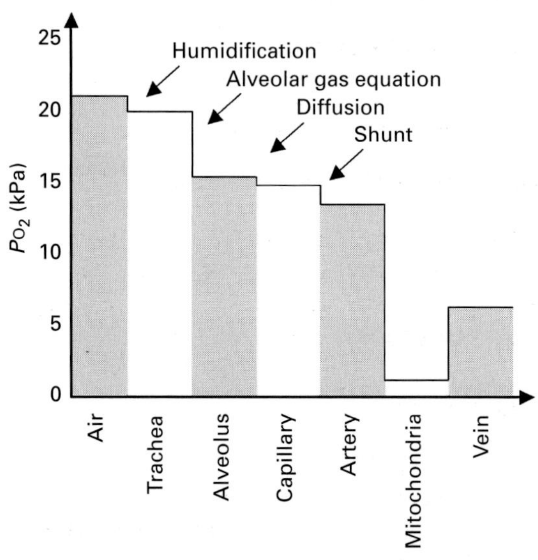

Stage	Process	Notes and equations
Air	–	$P\text{O}_2 = F\text{IO}_2.P_{\text{ATM}}$
Trachea	Humidification	$P\text{O}_2 = F\text{IO}_2(P_{\text{ATM}} - P\text{H}_2\text{O})$
Alveolus	Ventilation	$P\text{AO}_2 = [F\text{IO}_2(P_{\text{ATM}} - P\text{H}_2\text{O})] - (P\text{ACO}_2/\text{R})$
Capillary	Diffusion	Diffusion barrier negligible for O_2
Artery	Shunt, $\dot{V}/\dot{Q}$ mismatch	A–a gradient usually < 2 kPa
Mitochondria	–	Low $P\text{O}_2$ of around 1.5 kPa is usual
Veins	–	Normal $P\bar{v}\text{O}_2 = 6.3$ kPa

The delivery of any substance to an organ can be calculated if the concentration of the substance and the flow rate are measured.

$$D_{O_2} = CO.Ca_{O_2}.10$$

where D_{O_2} is delivery of O_2, CO is cardiac output and Ca_{O_2} is arterial O_2 content.

The multiplier 10 is used because Ca_{O_2} is measured in $ml.dl^{-1}$ whereas CO is measured in $l.min^{-1}$. The O_2 content of the blood is calculated using a specific equation that depends mainly on haemoglobin concentration, [Hb] and saturation (Sats).

$$Ca_{O_2} = (1.34[Hb]Sats) + (0.0225.Pa_{O_2})$$

if Pa_{O_2} is measured in kilopascals
or

$$Ca_{O_2} = (1.34[Hb]Sats) + (0.003.Pa_{O_2})$$

if Pa_{O_2} is measured in millimetres of mercury.

The number 1.34 is known as Hüffner's constant. It describes the volume of O_2 (ml) that can combine with each 1 g Hb. In vitro, its value is 1.39 but this becomes 1.34 in vivo because abnormal forms of Hb such as carboxyhaemoglobin and methaemoglobin are less able to carry O_2.

Supply and demand

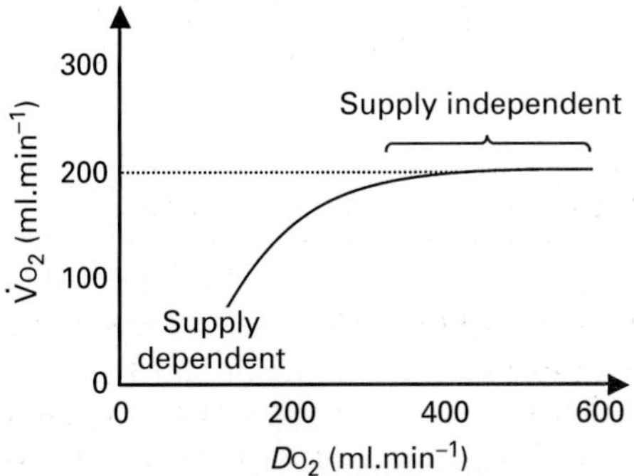

This curve demonstrates the relationship between oxygen delivery (D_{O_2}) and oxygen consumption ($\dot{V}_{O_2}$). The latter is normally around 200 $ml.min^{-1}$ and you should demonstrate that it is not affected until delivery falls to below approximately 300 $ml.min^{-1}$, which is known as critical D_{O_2}. When O_2 delivery is less than this, consumption becomes supply dependent. Above the critical value, it is termed supply independent.

The oxyhaemoglobin dissociation curve

The oxyhaemoglobin (oxy-Hb) dissociation curve is core knowledge for the examination and in clinical practice. You will be expected to have a very clear understanding and to be able to construct a very precise graph.

P_{50}

The partial pressure of O_2 in the blood at which haemoglobin is 50% saturated (kPa).

The oxyhaemoglobin dissociation curve

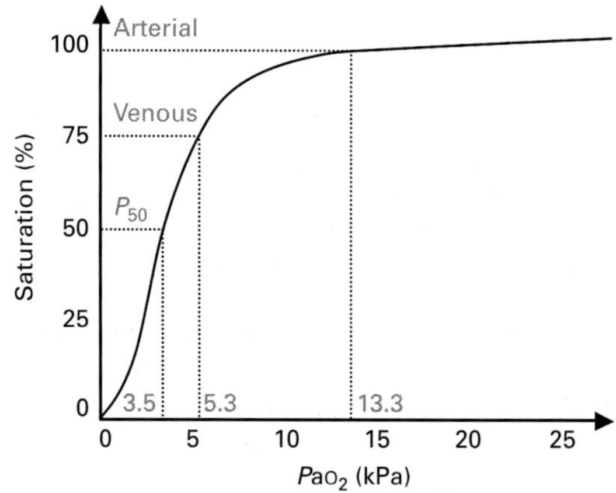

Draw and label the axes as shown; O_2 content can also be used on the *y* axis with a range of 0–21 ml.100 ml^{-1}. Your graph should accurately demonstrate three key points. The arterial point is plotted at 100% saturation and 13.3 kPa. The venous point is plotted at 75% saturation and 5.3 kPa. The P_{50} is plotted at 50% saturation (definition) and 3.5 kPa. Only when these three point are plotted should you draw in a smooth sigmoid curve that passes through all three. The curve is sigmoid because of the cooperative binding exhibited by Hb. In the deoxygenated state (deoxy-Hb), the Hb molecule is described as 'tense' and it is difficult for the first molecule of O_2 to bind. As O_2 binds to Hb the molecule relaxes (a conformational change occurs) and it become progressively easier for further molecules to bind. If asked to compare your curve with that of a different O_2 carrier such as myoglobin, draw a hyperbolic curve to the left of the original line. Myoglobin can only carry one O_2 molecule and so the curve does not have a sigmoid shape.

Factors affecting the curve

It is the change in position of the P_{50} that determines whether the curve has shifted to the left or to the right. You will be expected to be familiar with a number of factors that alter the position of the P_{50}.

Change in position of the P_{50}

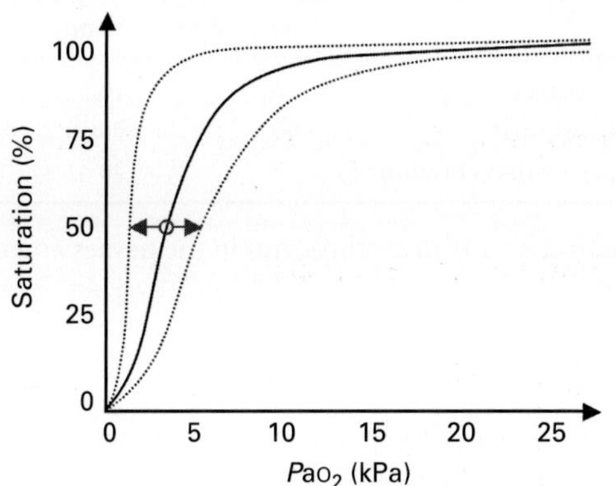

Left shift (increased affinity for O_2)	Right shift (decreased affinity for O_2)
Decreased $Paco_2$	Increased $Paco_2$
Alkalosis	Acidosis
Decreased temperature	Increased temperature
Decreased DPG	Increased DPG
Fetal haemoglobin	Pregnancy
Carbon monoxide	Altitude[a]
Methaemoglobin	Haemoglobin S

DPG, 2,3-diphosphoglycerate.
[a] High altitude can also cause a left shift of the P_{50} where Pao_2 is critically low.

The effect of pH on the affinity of Hb for O_2 is described as the Bohr effect.

The Bohr effect

> **The situation whereby the affinity of haemoglobin for oxygen is reduced by a reduction in pH and increased by an increase in pH.**

A decrease in pH results in a rightward shift of the curve and decreases the affinity of Hb for O_2. This tends to occur peripherally and allows the offloading of O_2 to the tissues. Conversely, in the lungs, the pH rises as CO_2 is offloaded and, therefore, O_2 affinity is increased to encourage uptake.

Carriage of carbon dioxide

Carbon dioxide is 20 times more soluble in blood than O_2 and is carried in three different forms.

	Arterial(%)	Venous(%)
Dissolved	5	10
Bicarbonate	90	60
Carbamino compounds	5	30

The following reaction occurs in erythrocytes in the tissues and explains how CO_2 is carried as HCO_3^-

$$CO_2 + H_2O \leftrightarrow H_2CO_3 \leftrightarrow H^+ + HCO_3^-$$

The reverse reaction occurs in the pulmonary capillaries.

The Haldane effect

The phenomenon by which deoxygenated haemoglobin is able to carry more CO_2 than oxygenated haemoglobin.

This occurs because deoxy-Hb forms carbamino-complexes with CO_2 more readily than oxy-Hb. Secondly, deoxy-Hb is a better buffer of H^+ than oxy-Hb and this increases the amount of HCO_3^- formed. Once formed, HCO_3^- diffuses out of the erythrocyte. To maintain electrical neutrality Cl^- moves in. This is known as the Cl^- shift or the Hamburger effect.

The Hamburger effect (chloride shift)

The transport of chloride ions into the cell as a result of outwards diffusion of bicarbonate in order to maintain electrical neutrality.

Dissociation of carbon dioxide versus oxygen

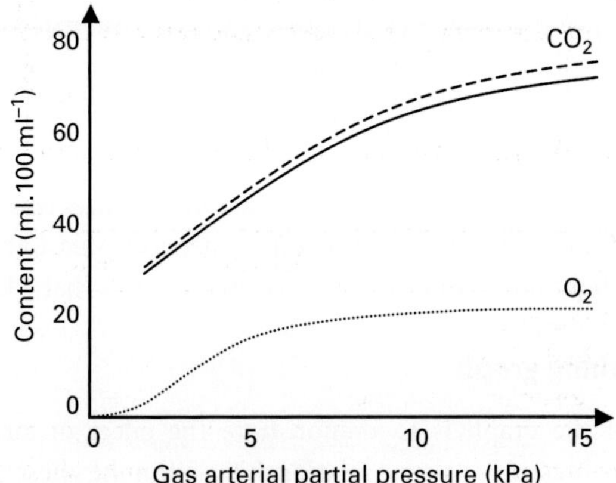

Carbon dioxide dissociation curves

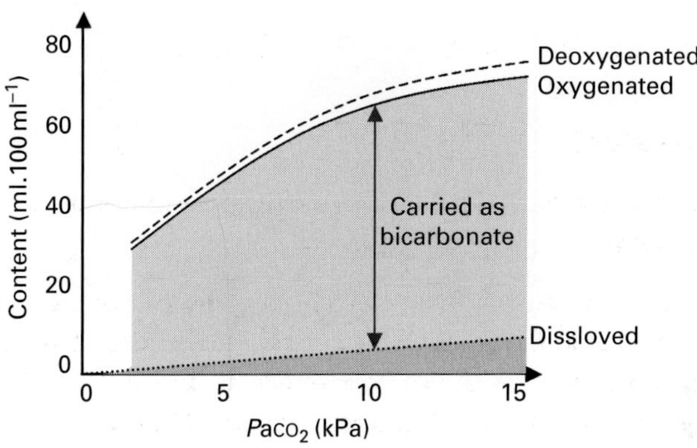

Dissolved The curve passes though the origin, rising as a shallow straight line as $P\text{aCO}_2$ rises.

Oxygenated The curve does not extend below 2 kPa as this lies outside the physiological range. It rises steeply at first before levelling off at approximately 60 ml.100 ml^{-1}.

Deoxygenated It is important to plot this line. At any $P\text{aCO}_2$, the CO_2 content will be higher than that of oxy-Hb. This is a graphical representation of the Haldane effect. As a result, the curve is plotted slightly above that of oxy-Hb. Be sure to point this relationship out to the examiner.

Other The amount of CO_2 lying between the dissolved line and the upper lines is that carried as HCO_3^-. The graph also demonstrates, therefore, that a greater percentage is carried as HCO_3^- in venous blood (area between deoxygenated and dissolved) than in arterial blood (area between oxygenated and dissolved).

Work of breathing

Work of breathing

In normal circumstances, the work done on expiration utilizes energy stored within the elastic tissues on inspiration. Expiration is, therefore, said to be passive unless the energy required to overcome airway resistance exceeds that which is stored.

Work of breathing graph

The purpose of the graph is to demonstrate the effect of airway and tissue resistance on the pressure–volume relationship within the chest.

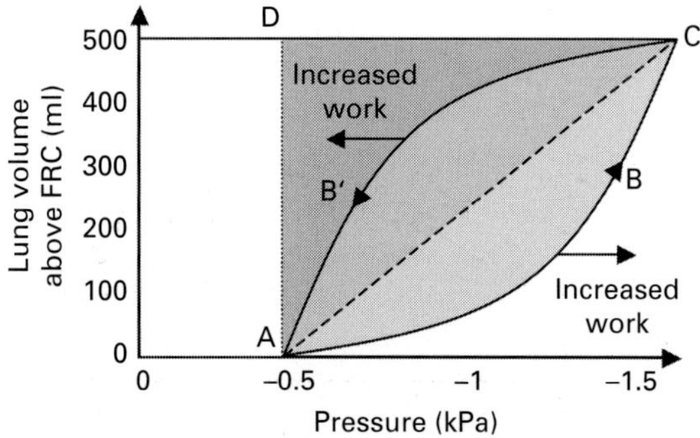

Draw and label the axes as shown. Remember the curve should only start to rise from −0.5 kPa on the *x* axis as the intrapleural pressure within the lung remains negative at tidal volumes. If there were no resistance to breathing, each tidal breath would increase its volume along the theoretical line AC and back again on expiration along the line CA.

Inspiration The line ABC is the physiological line traced on inspiration. The area ACDA represents work to overcome elastic tissues resistance. The extra area enclosed by ABCA represents the work done in overcoming viscous resistance and friction on inspiration. If this resistance increases, the curve bows to the right as shown.

Expiration The line CB′A is the physiological line traced on expiration. The area enclosed by CB′AC is the work done on expiration against airway resistance. As this area is enclosed within the area ACDA, the energy required can be supplied from the stored energy in the elastic tissues. If this resistance increases, the curve bows to the left, as shown. The difference in area between ACB′A and ACDA represents the energy lost as heat.

Control and effects of ventilation

You may be asked to draw the curves related to the control of ventilation or to the response of P_{ACO_2}/P_{AO_2} to changes in ventilation. It is important to be very clear about what question is being asked. The axes can be labelled in very similar ways but the curves are very different. There is no harm in asking for clarification in a viva setting before embarking on a description that may not be what the examiner is asking for.

Control of ventilation

Minute ventilation versus alveolar oxygen partial pressure

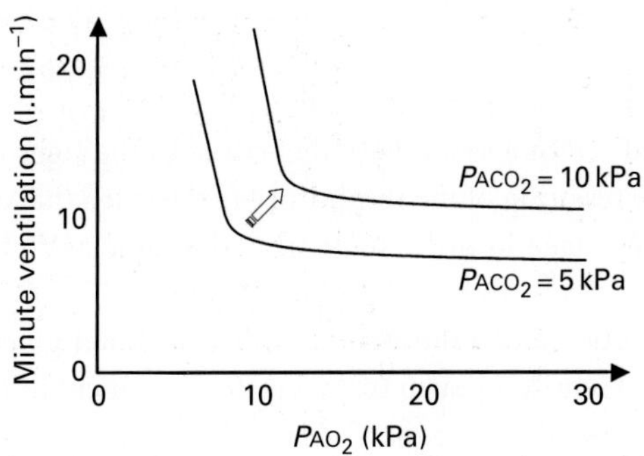

At P_{ACO_2} of 5 kPa The line should demonstrate that, under normal conditions, the minute volume (MV) remains relatively constant around 6 l.min^{-1} until the P_{AO_2} falls below 8 kPa. Show that the rise in MV following this is extremely steep. This illustrates the hypoxic drive, which is so often talked about in the setting of COPD.

At P_{ACO_2} of 10 kPa This line is plotted above and to the right of the first and demonstrates the effect of a coexisting hypercarbia on hypoxic ventilatory drive.

Minute ventilation versus alveolar carbon dioxide partial pressure

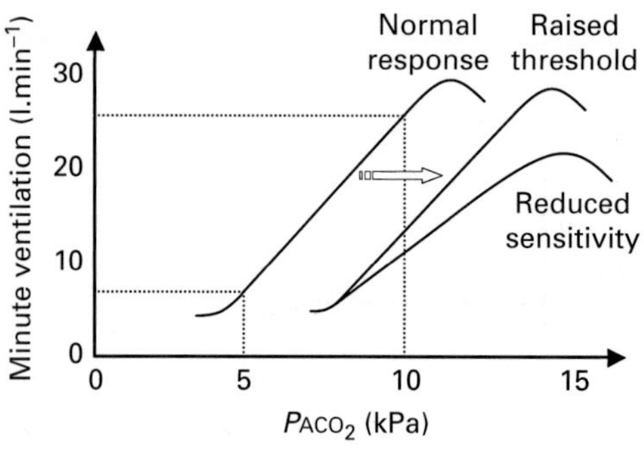

Normal Draw and label the axes as shown. Plot a normal $P\text{ACO}_2$ (5 kPa) at a normal MV ($6\,\text{l.min}^{-1}$). If the $P\text{ACO}_2$ is doubled, the MV increases four-fold in a linear fashion. Therefore, join the two points with a straight line. Above 10–11 kPa, the line should fall away, representing depression of respiration with very high $P\text{ACO}_2$. At the lower end of the line, the curve also flattens out and does not reach zero on either axis.

Raised threshold Plot a second parallel curve to the right of the first. This represents the resetting of the respiratory centre such that a higher $P\text{ACO}_2$ is required at any stage in order to achieve the same MV. This is seen with opiates.

Reduced sensitivity Plot a third curve with a shallower gradient. This represents decreased sensitivity such that a greater increment in $P\text{ACO}_2$ is required in order to achieve the same increment in MV. Also seen with opiates.

The following graphs deal with the effect that changes in ventilation have on the $P\text{ACO}_2$ or $P\text{AO}_2$, respectively. Make sure that you are clear about the differences between these graphs and the ones shown above.

Alveolar carbon dioxide partial pressure versus minute ventilation

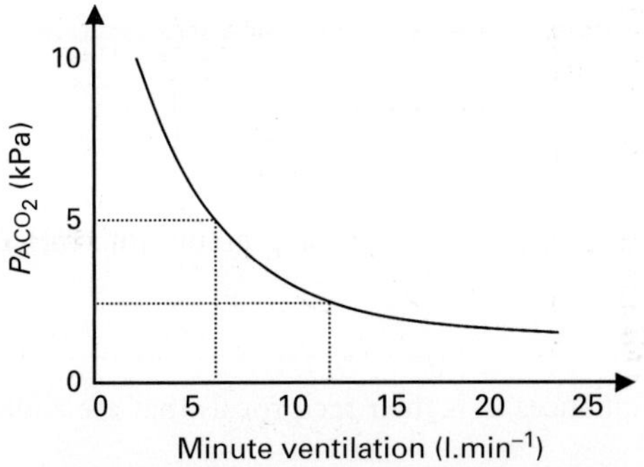

Draw and label the axes as shown. This graph demonstrates the effect that ventilation has on P_{ACO_2} rather than the control of ventilatory drive by CO_2 itself. As MV doubles, so the P_{ACO_2} halves. The curve is, therefore, a rectangular hyperbola. Begin by plotting a normal P_{ACO_2} (5 kPa) at a normal MV (6 l.min^{-1}). Draw one or two more points at which MV has doubled (or quadrupled) and P_{ACO_2} has halved (or quartered). Finish by drawing a smooth curve through all the points you have drawn.

Alveolar oxygen partial pressure versus minute ventilation

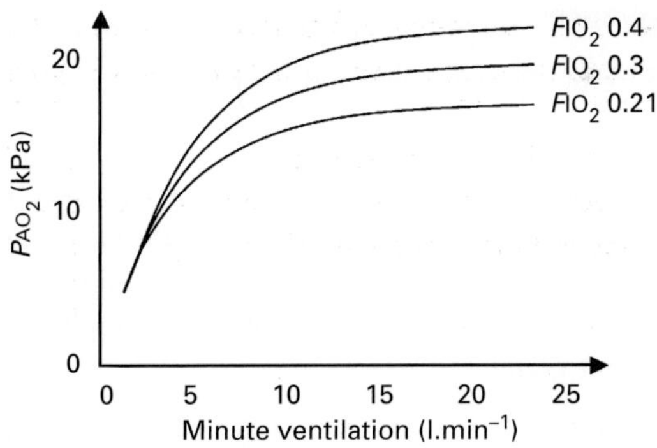

Draw and label the axes as shown. This graph demonstrates the effect of ventilation on P_{AO_2}. Start by marking a point at a normal MV of 6 l.min^{-1} and a normal P_{AO_2} of 13.3 kPa. Draw a hyperbolic curve passing through this point just before flattening out. It should not pass through the origin as this is unphysiological. The curve illustrates how large increases in MV have little effect on P_{AO_2}. The only reliable way to increase the P_{AO_2} is to increase the F_{IO_2}, which is demonstrated by drawing additional parallel curves as shown.

Compliance and resistance

Compliance

The volume change per unit change in pressure ($ml.cmH_2O^{-1}$ or $l.kPa^{-1}$).

Lung compliance

When adding compliances, it is their reciprocals that are added (as with capacitance) so that:

$$1/C_{TOTAL} = (1/C_{CHEST}) + (1/C_{LUNG})$$

where C_{CHEST} is chest compliance (1.5–2.0 $l.kPa^{-1}$ or 150–200 $ml.cmH_2O^{-1}$), C_{LUNG} is lung compliance (1.5–2 $l.kPa^{-1}$ or 150–200 $ml.cmH_2O^{-1}$) and C_{TOTAL} is total compliance (7.5–10.0 $l.kPa^{-1}$ or 75–100 $ml.cmH_2O^{-1}$).

Static compliance

The compliance of the lung measured when all gas flow has ceased ($ml.cmH_2O^{-1}$ or $l.kPa^{-1}$).

Dynamic compliance

The compliance of the lung measured during the respiratory cycle when gas flow is still ongoing ($ml.cmH_2O^{-1}$ or $l.kPa^{-1}$)

Static compliance is usually higher than dynamic compliance because there is time for volume and pressure equilibration between the lungs and the measuring system. The measured volume tends to increase and the measured pressure tends to decrease, both of which act to increase compliance. Compliance is often plotted on a pressure–volume graph.

Resistance

The pressure change per unit change in volume ($cmH_2O.ml^{-1}$ or $kPa.l^{-1}$).

Lung resistance

When adding resistances, they are added as normal integers (as with electrical resistance)

$$\text{Total resistance} = \text{Chest wall resistance} + \text{lung resistance}$$

Whole lung pressure–volume loop

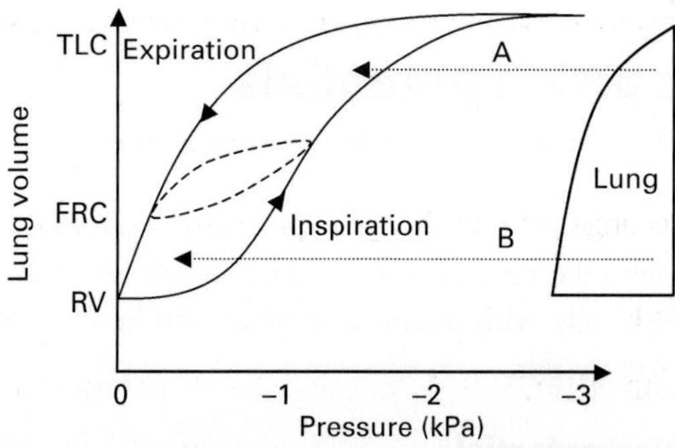

This graph can be used to explain a number of different aspects of compliance. The axes as shown are for spontaneous ventilation as the pressure is negative. The curve for compliance during mechanical ventilation looks the same but the *x* axis should be labelled with positive pressures. The largest curve should be drawn first to represent a vital capacity breath.

Inspiration The inspiratory line is sigmoid and, therefore, initially flat as negative pressure is needed before a volume change will take place. The mid segment is steepest around FRC and the end segment is again flat as the lungs are maximally distended and so poorly compliant in the face of further pressure change.

Expiration The expiratory limb is a smooth curve. At high lung volumes, the compliance is again low and the curve flat. The steep part of the curve is around FRC as pressure returns to baseline.

Tidal breath To demonstrate the compliance of the lung during tidal ventilation, draw the dotted curve. This curve is similar in shape to the first but the volume change is smaller. It should start from, and end at, the FRC by definition.

Regional differences You can also demonstrate that alveoli at the top of the lung lie towards the top of the compliance curve, as shown by line A. They are already distended by traction on the lung from below and so are less compliant for a given pressure change than those lower down. Alveoli at the bottom of the lung lie towards the bottom of the curve, as shown by line B. For a given pressure change they are able to distend more and so their compliance is greater. With mechanical ventilation, both points move down the curve, resulting in the upper alveoli becoming more compliant.

Cardiac action potentials

General definitions relating to action potentials are given in Section 9. This section deals specifically with action potentials within the cardiac pacemaker cells and conducting system.

Pacemaker action potential

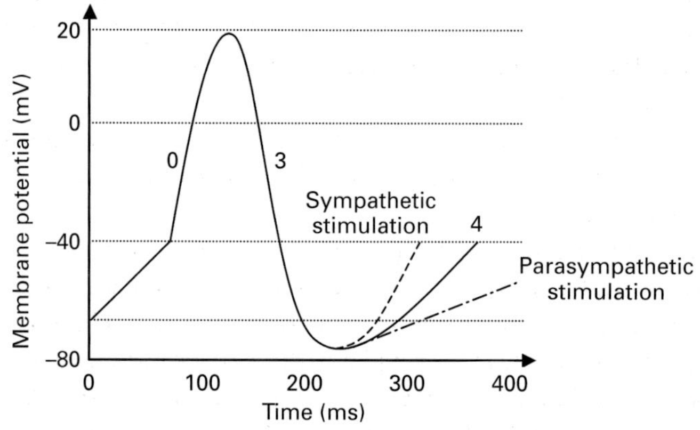

Phase 0 Spontaneous 'baseline drift' results in the threshold potential being achieved at – 40 mV. Slow L-type Ca^{2+} channels are responsible for further depolarization so you should ensure that you demonstrate a relatively slurred upstroke owing to slow Ca^{2+} influx.

Phase 3 Repolarization occurs as Ca^{2+} channels close and K^+ channels open. Efflux of K^+ from within the cell repolarizes the cell fairly rapidly compared with Ca^{2+}-dependent depolarization.

Phase 4 Hyperpolarization occurs before K^+ efflux has completely stopped and is followed by a gradual drift towards threshold (pacemaker) potential. This is reflects a Na^+ leak, T-type Ca^{2+} channels and a Na^+/Ca^{2+} pump, which all encourage cations to enter the cell. The slope of your line during phase 4 is altered by sympathetic (increased gradient) and parasympathetic (decreased gradient) nervous system activity.

Cardiac conduction system action potential

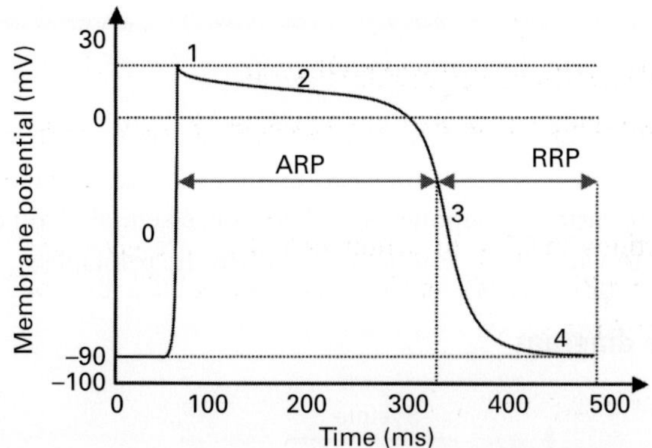

Phase 0 Rapid depolarization occurs after threshold potential is reached owing to fast Na^+ influx. The gradient of this line should be almost vertical as shown.

Phase 1 Repolarization begins to occur as Na^+ channels close and K^+ channels open. Phase 1 is short in duration and does not cause repolarization below 0 mV.

Phase 2 A plateau occurs owing to the opening of L-type Ca^{2+} channels, which offset the action of K^+ channels and maintain depolarization. During this phase, no further depolarization is possible. This is an important point to demonstrate and explains why tetany is not possible in cardiac muscle. This time period is the absolute refractory period (ARP). The plateau should not be drawn completely horizontal as repolarization is slowed by Ca^{2+} channels but not halted altogether.

Phase 3 The L-type Ca^{2+} channels close and K^+ efflux now causes repolarization as seen before. The relative refractory period (RRP) occurs during phases 3 and 4.

Phase 4 The Na^+/K^+ pump restores the ionic gradients by pumping $3Na^+$ out of the cell in exchange for $2K^+$. The overall effect is, therefore, the slow loss of positive ionic charge from within the cell.

The cardiac cycle

The key point of the cardiac cycle diagram is to be able to use it to explain the flow of blood through the left side of the heart and into the aorta. An appreciation of the timing of the various components is, therefore, essential if you are to draw an accurate diagram with which you hope to explain the principle.

Cardiac cycle diagram

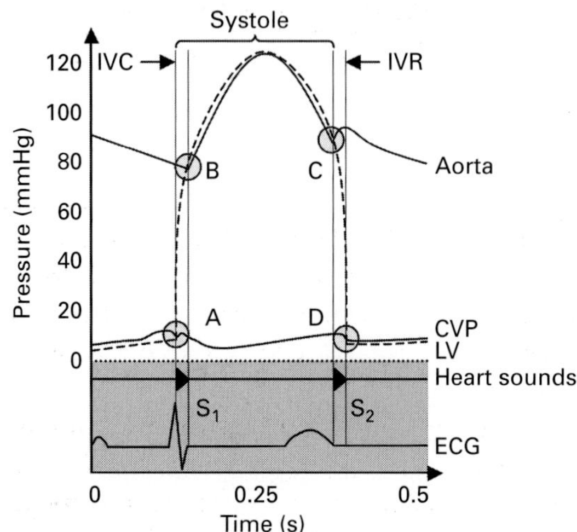

Timing reference curves

Electrocardiography It may be easiest to begin with an ECG trace. Make sure that the trace is drawn widely enough so that all the other curves can be plotted without appearing too cramped. The ECG need only be a stylized representation but is key in pinning down the timing of all the other curves.

Heart sounds Sound S_1 occurs at the beginning of systole as the mitral and tricuspid valves close; S_2 occurs at the beginning of diastole as the aortic and pulmonary valves close. These points should be in line with the beginning of electrical depolarization (QRS) and the end of repolarization (T), respectively, on the ECG trace. The duration of S_1 matches the duration of isovolumic contraction (IVC) and that of S_2 matches that of isovolumic relaxation (IVR). Mark the vertical lines on the plot to demonstrate this fact.

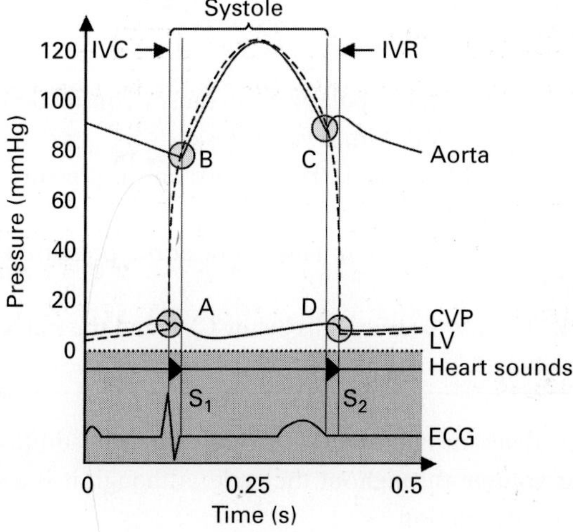

Pressure curves

Central venous pressure (CVP) The usual CVP trace should be drawn on at a pressure of 5–10 mmHg. The 'c' wave occurs during IVC owing to bulging of the closed tricuspid as the ventricle begins to contract. The 'y' descent occurs immediately following IVR as the tricuspid valve opens and allows free flow of blood into the near empty ventricle.

Left Ventricle (LV) A simple inverted 'U' curve is drawn that has its baseline between 0 and 5 mmHg and its peak at 120 mmHg. During diastole, its pressure must be less than that of the CVP to enable forward flow. It only increases above CVP during systole. The curve between points A and B demonstrates why the initial contraction is isovolumic. The LV pressure is greater than CVP so the mitral valve must be closed, but it is less than aortic pressure so the aortic valve must also be closed. The same is true of the curve between points C and D with regards to IVR.

Aorta A familiar arterial pressure trace. Its systolic component follows the LV trace between points B and C at a slightly lower pressure to enable forward flow. During IVR, closure of the aortic valve and bulging of the sinus of Valsalva produce the dicrotic notch, after which the pressure falls to its diastolic value.

Important timing points

A	Start of IVC. Electrical depolarization causes contraction and the LV pressure rises above CVP. Mitral valve closes (S_1).
B	End of IVC. The LV pressure rises above aortic pressure. Aortic valve opens and blood flows into the circulation.
C	Start of IVR. The LV pressure falls below aortic pressure and the aortic valve closes (S_2).
D	End of IVR. The LV pressure falls below CVP and the mitral valve opens. Ventricular filling.

The cardiac cycle diagram is sometimes plotted with the addition of a curve to show ventricular volume throughout the cycle. Although it is a simple curve, it can reveal a lot of information.

Left ventricular volume curve

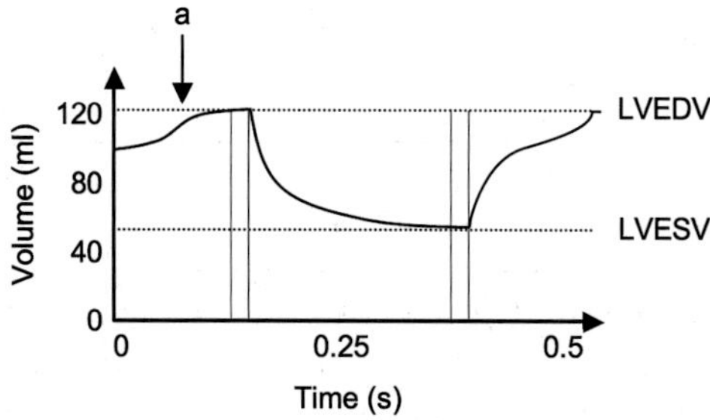

This trace shows the volume of the left ventricle throughout the cycle. The important point is the atrial kick seen at point a. Loss of this kick in atrial fibrillation and other conditions can adversely affect cardiac function through impaired LV filling. The maximal volume occurs at the end of diastolic filling and is labelled the left ventricular end-diastolic volume (LVEDV). In the same way, the minimum volume is the left ventricular end-systolic volume (LVESV). The difference between these two values must, therefore, be the stroke volume (SV), which is usually 70 ml as demonstrated above. The ejection fraction (EF) is the SV as a percentage of the LVEDV and is around 60% in the diagram above.

Pressure and flow calculations

Mean arterial pressure

$$MAP = \frac{SBP + (2\,DBP)}{3}$$

or

$$MAP = DBP + (PP/3)$$

MAP is mean arterial pressure, SBP is systolic blood pressure, DBP is diastolic blood pressure and PP is pulse pressure.

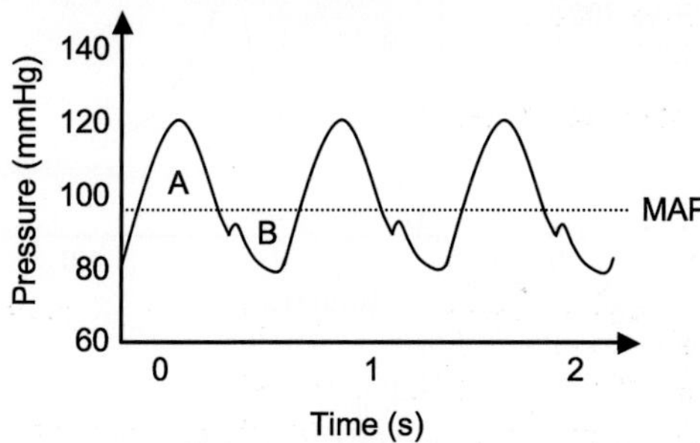

Draw and label the axes as shown. Draw a sensible looking arterial waveform between values of 120 and 80 mmHg. The numerical MAP given by the above equations is 93 mmHg, so mark your MAP line somewhere around this value. The point of the graph is to demonstrate that the MAP is the line which makes area A equal to area B

Coronary perfusion pressure

The maximum pressure of the blood perfusing the coronary arteries (mmHg).

or

The pressure difference between the aortic diastolic pressure and the LVEDP (mmHg).

So

$$CPP = ADP - LVEDP$$

CPP is coronary perfusion pressure and ADP is aortic diastolic pressure.

Coronary blood flow

Coronary blood flow reflects the balance between pressure and resistance

$$CBF = \frac{CPP}{CVR}$$

CBF is coronary blood flow, CPP is coronary perfusion pressure and CVR is coronary vascular resistance.

Coronary perfusion pressure is measured during diastole as the pressure gradient between ADP and LVEDP is greatest during this time. This means that CBF is also greatest during diastole, especially in those vessels supplying the high-pressure left ventricle. The trace below represents the flow within such vessels.

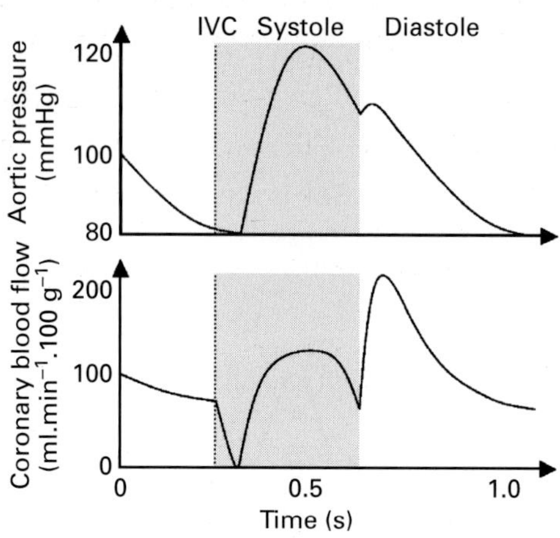

Draw and label two sets of axes so that you can show waveforms for both aortic pressure and coronary blood flow. Start by marking on the zones for systole and diastole as shown. Remember from the cardiac cycle that systole actually begins with isovolumic contraction of the ventricle. Mark this line on both graphs. Next plot an aortic pressure waveform remembering that the pressure does not rise during IVC as the aortic valve is closed at this point. A dicrotic notch occurs at the start of diastole and the cycle repeats. The CBF is approximately 100 $ml.min^{-1}.100\,g^{-1}$ at the end of diastole but rapidly falls to zero during IVC owing to direct compression of the coronary vessels and a huge rise in intraventricular pressure. During systole, CBF rises above its previous level as the aortic pressure is higher and the ventricular wall tension is slightly reduced. The shape of your curve at this point should roughly follow that of the aortic pressure waveform during systole. The key point to demonstrate is that it is not until diastole occurs that perfusion rises substantially. During diastole, ventricular wall tension is low and so the coronaries are not directly compressed. In addition, intraventricular pressure is low and aortic pressure is high in the early stages and so the perfusion pressure is maximized. As the right ventricle (RV) is a low-pressure/tension ventricle compared with the left, CBF continues throughout systole and diastole without falling to zero. Right CBF ranges between 5 and 15 $ml.min^{-1}.100\,g^{-1}$. The general shape of the trace is otherwise similar to that of the left.

Central venous pressure

The central venous pressure is the hydrostatic pressure generated by the blood in the great veins. It can be used as a surrogate of right atrial pressure (mmHg).

The CVP waveform should be very familiar to you. You will be expected to be able to draw and label the trace below and discuss how the waveform may change with different pathologies.

Central venous pressure waveform

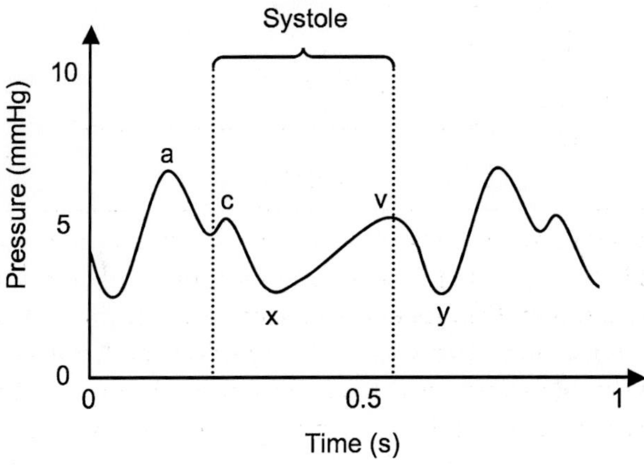

The a wave This is caused by atrial contraction and is, therefore, seen before the carotid pulsation. It is absent in atrial fibrillation and abnormally large if the atrium is hypertrophied, for example with tricuspid stenosis. 'Cannon' waves caused by atrial contraction against a closed tricuspid valve would also occur at this point. If such waves are regular they reflect a nodal rhythm, and if irregular they are caused by complete heart block.

The c wave This results from the bulging of the tricuspid valve into the right atrium during ventricular contraction.

The v wave This results from atrial filling against a closed tricuspid valve. Giant v waves are caused by tricuspid incompetence and these mask the 'x' descent.

The x descent The fall at x is caused by downward movement of the heart during ventricular systole and relaxation of the atrium.

The y descent The fall at y is caused by passive ventricular filling after opening of the tricuspid valve.

Pulmonary arterial wedge pressure

The pulmonary artery wedge pressure (PAWP) is an indirect estimate of left atrial pressure. A catheter passes through the right side of the heart into the pulmonary vessels and measures changing pressures. After the catheter has been inserted, a balloon at its tip is inflated, which helps it to float through the heart chambers. It is possible to measure all the right heart pressures and the pulmonary artery occlusion pressure (PAOP). The PAOP should ideally be measured with the catheter tip in west zone 3 of the lung. This is where the pulmonary artery pressure is greater than both the alveolar pressure and pulmonary venous pressure, ensuring a continuous column of blood to the left atrium throughout the respiratory cycle. The PAOP may be used as a surrogate of the left atrial pressure and, therefore, LVEDP. However, pathological conditions may easily upset this relationship.

Pulmonary arterial wedge pressure waveform

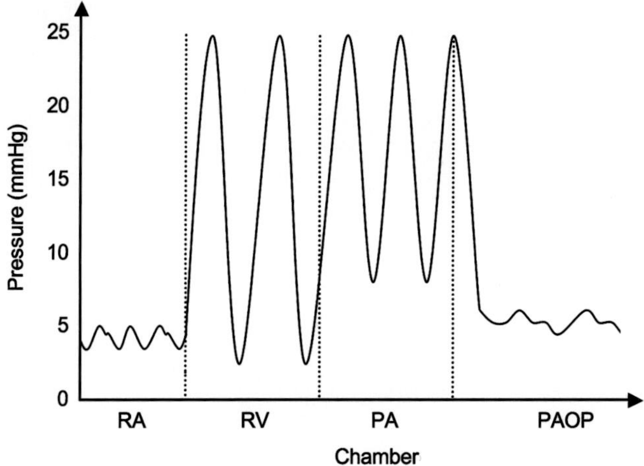

Right atrium (RA) The pressure waveform is identical to the CVP. The normal pressure is 0–5 mmHg.

Right ventricle (RV) The RV pressure waveform should oscillate between 0–5 mmHg and 20–25 mmHg.

Pulmonary atery (PA) As the catheter moves into the PA, the diastolic pressure will increase owing to the presence of the pulmonary valve. Normal PA systolic pressure is the same as the RV systolic pressure but the diastolic pressure rises to 10–15 mmHg.

PAOP This must be lower than the PA diastolic pressure to ensure forward flow. It is drawn as an undulating waveform similar to the CVP trace. The normal value is 6–12 mmHg. The values vary with the respiratory cycle and are read at the end of expiration. In spontaneously ventilating patients, this will be the highest reading and in mechanically ventilated patients, it will be the lowest. The PAOP is found at an insertion length of around 45 cm.

The Frank–Starling relationship

Before considering the relationship itself, it may be useful to recap on a few of the salient definitions.

Cardiac output

$$CO = SV \times HR$$

where CO is cardiac output, SV is stroke volume and HR is heart rate.

Stroke volume

The volume of blood ejected from the left ventricle with every contraction (ml).

Stroke volume is itself dependent on the prevailing preload, afterload and contractility.

Preload

The initial length of the cardiac muscle fibre before contraction begins.

This can be equated to the end-diastolic volume and is described by the Frank–Starling mechanism. Clinically it is equated to the CVP when studying the RV or the PAOP when studying the LV.

Pulmonary artery occlusion pressure.

Afterload

The tension which needs to be generated in cardiac muscle fibres before shortening will occur.

Although not truly analogous, afterload is often clinically equated to the systemic vascular resistance (SVR).

Contractility

The intrinsic ability of cardiac muscle fibres to do work with a given preload and afterload.

Preload and afterload are extrinsic factors that influence contractility whereas intrinsic factors include autonomic nervous system activity and catecholamine effects.

Frank–Starling law

The strength of cardiac contraction is dependent upon the initial fibre length.

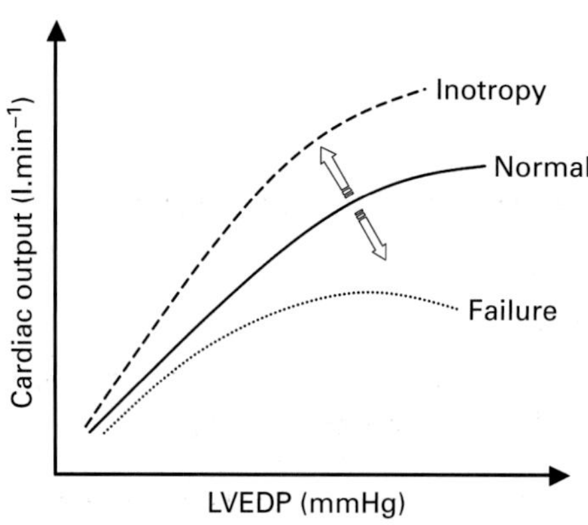

Normal The LVEDP may be used as a measure of preload or 'initial fibre length'. Cardiac output increases as LVEDP increases until a maximum is reached. This is because there is an optimal degree of overlap of the muscle filaments and increasing the fibre length increases the effective overlap and, therefore, contraction.

Inotropy Draw this curve above and to the left of the 'normal' curve. This positioning demonstrates that, for any given LVEDP, the resultant cardiac output is greater.

Failure Draw this curve below and to the right of the 'normal' curve. Highlight the fall in cardiac output at high LVEDP by drawing a curve that falls back towards baseline at these values. This occurs when cardiac muscle fibres are overstretched. The curve demonstrates that, at any given LVEDP, the cardiac output is less and the maximum cardiac output is reduced, and that the cardiac output can be adversely affected by rises in LVEDP which would be beneficial in the normal heart.

Changes in inotropy will move the curve up or down as described above. Changes in volume status will move the status of an individual heart along the curve it is on.

Venous return and capillary dynamics

Venous return

Venous return will depend on pressure relations:

$$VR = \frac{(MSFP - RAP)}{R_{ven}} \times 80$$

where VR is venous return, MSFP is mean systemic filling pressure, RAP is right atrial pressure and R_{ven} is venous resistance.

The MSFP is the weighted average of the pressures in all parts of the systemic circulation.

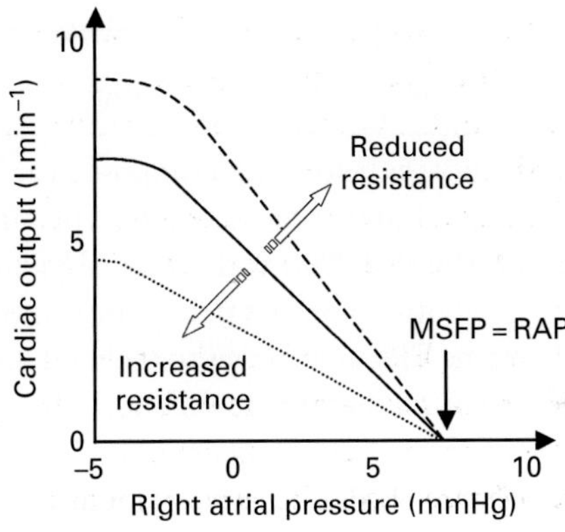

Draw and label the axes as shown. Venous return depends on a pressure gradient being in place along the vessel. Consider the situation where the pressure in the RA is was equal to the MSFP. No pressure gradient exists and so no flow will occur. Venous return must, therefore, be zero. This would normally occur at a RAP of approximately 7 mmHg. As RAP falls, flow increases, so draw your middle (normal) line back towards the *y* axis in a linear fashion. At approximately −4 mmHg, the extrathoracic veins tend to collapse and so a plateau of venous return is reached, which you should demonstrate. Lowering the resistance in the venous system increases the venous return and, therefore, the cardiac output. This can be shown by drawing a line with a steeper gradient. The opposite is also true and can similarly be demonstrated on the graph. Changes in MSFP will shift the intercept of the line with the *x* axis.

Changes to the venous return curve

The slope and the intercept of the VR curve on the x axis can be altered as described above. Although it is unlikely that your questioning will proceed this far, it may be useful to have an example of how this may be relevant clinically.

Increased filling

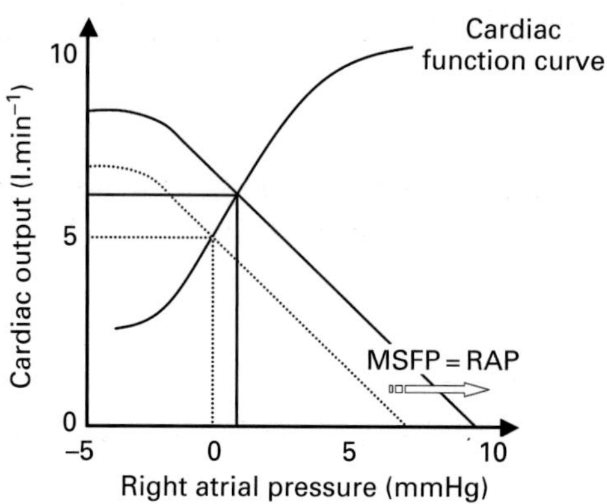

Construct a normal VR curve as before. Superimpose a cardiac function curve (similar to the Starling curve) so that the lines intercept at a cardiac output of 5 l.min^{-1} and a RAP of 0 mmHg. This is the normal intercept and gives the input pressure (RAP) and output flow (CO) for a normal ventricle. If MSFP is now increased by filling, the VR curve moves to the right so that RAP = MSFP at 10 mmHg. The intercept on the cardiac function curve has now changed. The values are unimportant but you should demonstrate that the CO and RAP have both increased for this ventricle by virtue of filling.

Altered venous resistance

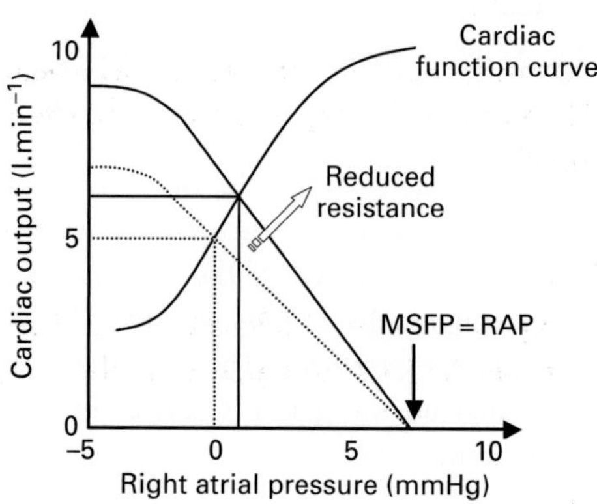

Construct your normal curves as before. This time the patient's systemic resistance has been lowered by a factor such as anaemia (reduced viscosity) or drug administration (vessel dilatation). Assuming that the MSFP remains the same, which may require fluid administration to counteract vessel dilatation, the CO and RAP for this ventricle will increase. Demonstrate that changes in resistance alter the slope of your line rather than the 'pivot point' on the *x* axis.

Capillary dynamics

As well as his experiments on the heart, Starling proposed a physiological explanation for fluid movement across the capillaries. It depends on the understanding of four key terms.

Capillary hydrostatic pressure

The pressure exerted on the capillary by a column of whole blood within it (P_c; mmHg).

Interstitial hydrostatic pressure

The pressure exerted on the capillary by the fluid which surrounds it in the interstitial space (P_i; mmHg).

Capillary oncotic pressure

The pressure that would be required to prevent the movement of water across a semipermeable membrane owing to the osmotic effect of large plasma proteins. (π_c; mmHg).

Interstitial osmotic pressure

The pressure that would be required to prevent the movement of water across a semipermeable membrane owing to the osmotic effect of interstitial fluid particles (π_i; mmHg).

Fluid movement

The ratios of these four pressures alter at different areas of the capillary network so that net fluid movement into or out of the capillary can also change as shown below.

$$\text{Net filtration pressure} = \text{Outward forces} - \text{Inward forces}$$
$$= K[(P_c + \pi_i) - (P_i + \pi_c)]$$

where K is the capillary filtration coefficient and reflects capillary permeability.

Arteriolar end of capillary

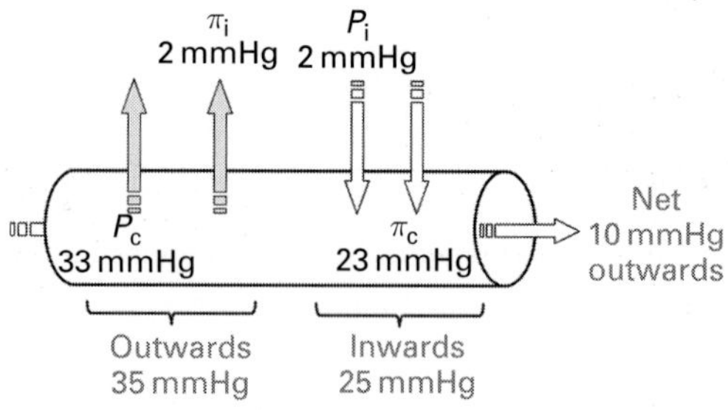

Centre region of capillary

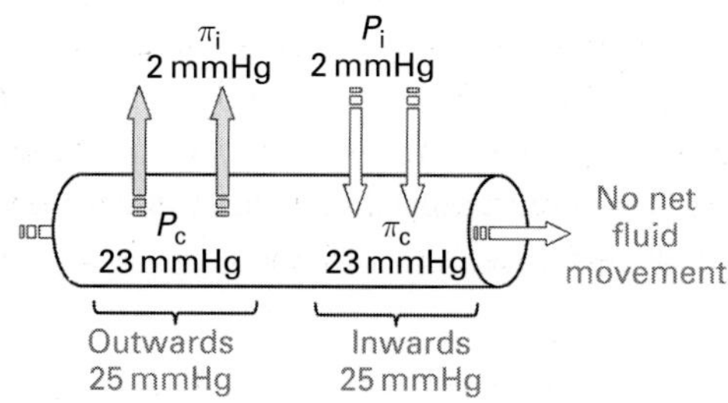

Venular end of capillary

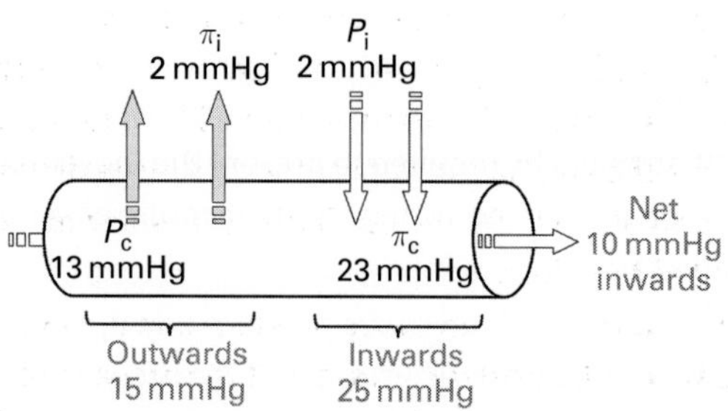

The precise numbers you choose to use are not as important as the concept that, under normal circumstances, the net filtration and absorptive forces are the same. Anything which alters these component pressures such as venous congestion (P_c increased) or dehydration loss (π_c increased) will, in turn, shift the balance towards filtration or absorption, respectively. You should have some examples ready to discuss.

The above information may also be demonstrated on a graph, which can help to explain how changes in vascular tone can alter the amount of fluid filtered or reabsorbed.

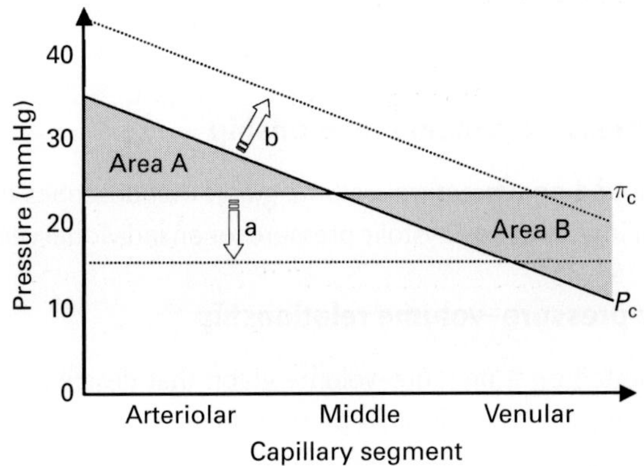

Draw and label the axes and mark a horizontal line at a pressure of 23 mmHg to represent the constant π_c. Next draw a line sloping downwards from left to right from 35 mmHg to 15 mmHg to represent the falling capillary hydrostatic pressure (P_c). Area A represents the fluid filtered out of the capillary on the arteriolar side and area B represents that which is reabsorbed on the venous side. Normally these two areas are equal and there is no net loss or gain of fluid.

Arrow a This represents a fall in π_c; area A, therefore, becomes much larger than area B, indicating overall net filtration of fluid out of the vasculature. This may be caused by hypoalbuminaemia and give rise to oedema.

Arrow b This represents an increased P_c. If only the arteriolar pressure rises, the gradient of the line will increase, whereas if the venous pressure rises in tandem the line will undergo a parallel shift. The net result is again filtration. This occurs clinically in vasodilatation. The opposite scenario is seen in shock, where the arterial pressure at the capillaries drops. This results in net reabsorption of fluid into the capillaries and is one of the compensatory mechanisms to blood loss.

Other features An increase in venous pressure owing to venous congestion will increase venous hydrostatic pressure. If the pressure on the arterial side of the capillaries is unchanged, this moves the venous end of the hydrostatic pressure line upwards and the gradient of the line decreases. This increases area A and decreases area B, again leading to net filtration.

Ventricular pressure–volume relationship

Graphs of ventricular (systolic) pressure versus volume are very useful tools and can be used to demonstrate a number of principles related to cardiovascular physiology.

End-systolic pressure–volume relationship

The line plotted on a pressure–volume graph that describes the relationship between filling status and systolic pressure for an individual ventricle (ESPVR).

End-diastolic pressure–volume relationship

The line plotted on a pressure–volume graph that describes the relationship between filling status and diastolic pressure for an individual ventricle (EDPVR).

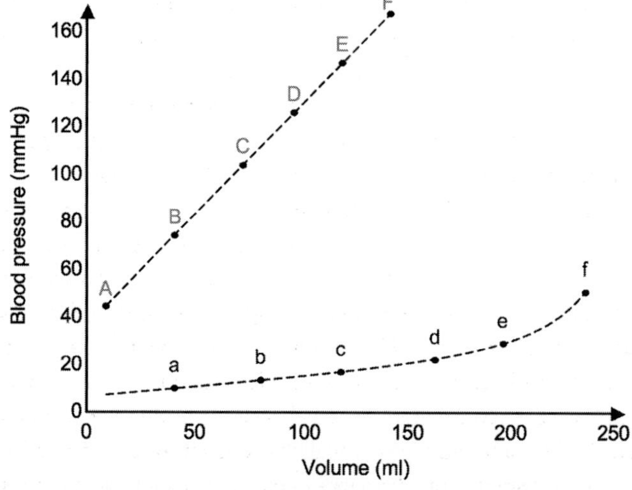

A–F This straight line represents the ESPVR. If a ventricle is taken and filled to volume 'a', it will generate pressure 'A' at the end of systole. When filled to volume 'b' it will generate pressure 'B' and so on. Each ventricle will have a curve specific to its overall function but a standard example is shown below. Changes in contractility can alter the gradient of the line.

a–f This curve represents the EDPVR. When the ventricle is filled to volume 'a' it will, by definition, have an end-diastolic pressure 'a'. When filled to volume 'b' it will have a pressure 'b' and so on. The line offers some information about diastolic function and is altered by changes in compliance, distensibility and relaxation of the ventricle.

Pressure–volume relationship

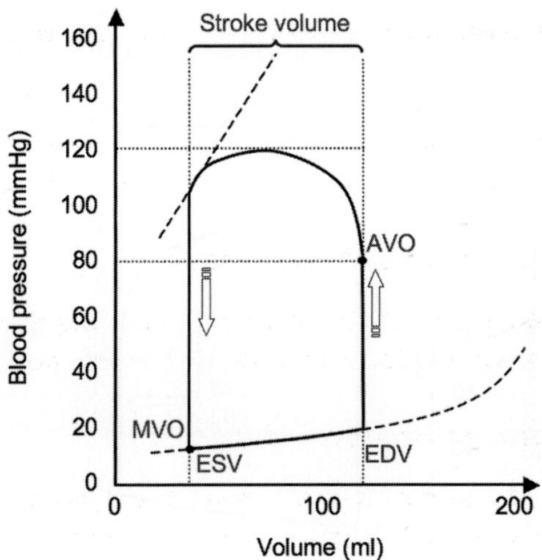

After drawing and labelling the axes as shown, plot sample ESPVR and EDPVR curves (dotted). It is easiest to draw the curve in an anti-clockwise direction starting from a point on the EDPVR that represents the EDV. A normal value for EDV may be 120 ml. The initial upstroke is vertical as this is a period of isovolumic contraction during early systole. The aortic valve opens (AVO) when ventricular pressure exceeds aortic diastolic pressure (80 mmHg). Ejection then occurs and the ventricular blood volume decreases as the pressure continues to rise towards systolic (120 mmHg) before tailing off. The curve should cross the ESPVR line at a point *after* peak systolic pressure has been attained. The volume ejected during this period of systole is the SV and is usually in the region of 70 ml. During early diastole, there is an initial period of isovolumic relaxation, which is demonstrated as another vertical line. When the ventricular pressure falls below the atrial pressure, the mitral valve opens (MVO) and blood flows into the ventricle so expanding its volume prior to the next contraction. The area contained within this loop represents the external work of the ventricle (work = pressure × volume).

Ejection fraction

The percentage of ventricular volume that is ejected from the ventricle during systolic contraction: (%)

$$EF = \frac{EDV - ESV}{EDV} \times 100$$

where EF is ejection fraction, EDV is end-diastolic volume, ESV is end-systolic volume and (EDV – ESV) is stroke volume.

Increased preload

Although an isolated increase in preload is unlikely to occur physiologically, it is useful to have an idea of how such a situation would affect your curve.

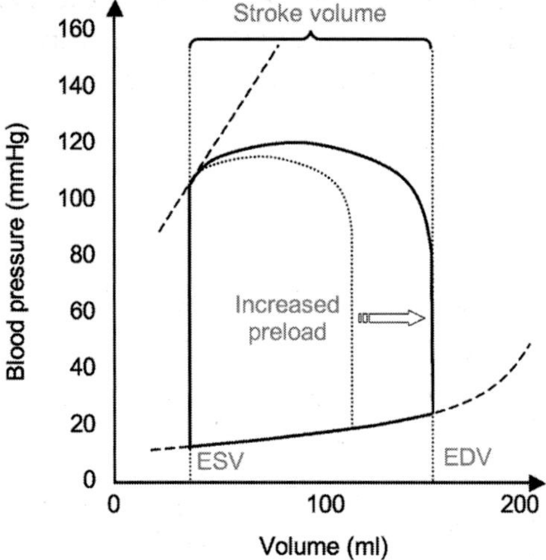

Based on the previous diagram, a pure increase in preload will move the EDV point to the right by virtue of increased filling during diastole. This will widen the loop and thus increase the stroke work. As a consequence, the SV is also increased. Note that the end systolic pressure (ESP) and the ESV remain unchanged in the diagram above. Under physiological conditions these would both increase, with the effect of moving the whole curve up and to the right.

Increased afterload

Again, increased afterload is non-physiological but it helps with understanding during discussion of the topic.

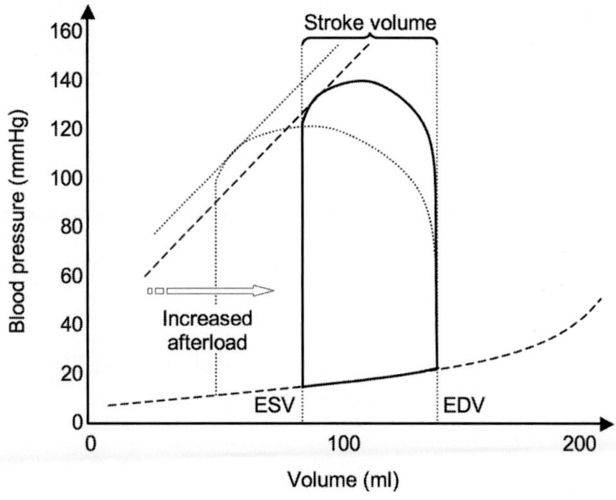

A pure increase in afterload will move the ESPVR line and thus the ESV point to the right by virtue of reduced emptying during systole. Emptying is curtailed because the ventricle is now ejecting against an increased resistance. As such, the ejection phase does not begin until a higher pressure is reached (here about 100 mmHg) within the ventricle. The effect is to create a tall, narrow loop with a consequent reduction in SV and similar or slightly reduced stroke work.

Altered contractility

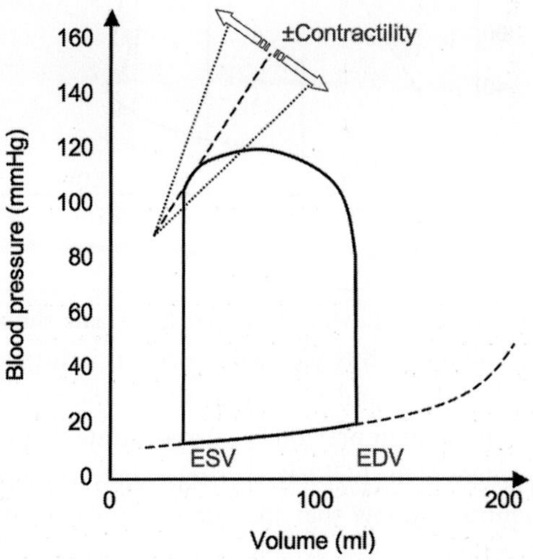

A pure increase in contractility shifts the ESPVR line up and to the left. The EDV is unaltered but the ESV is reduced and, therefore, the EF increases. The loop is wider and so the SV and work are both increased. A reduction in contractility has the opposite effect.

The failing ventricle

Diastolic function depends upon the compliance, distensibility and relaxation of the ventricle. All three aspects combine to alter the curve.

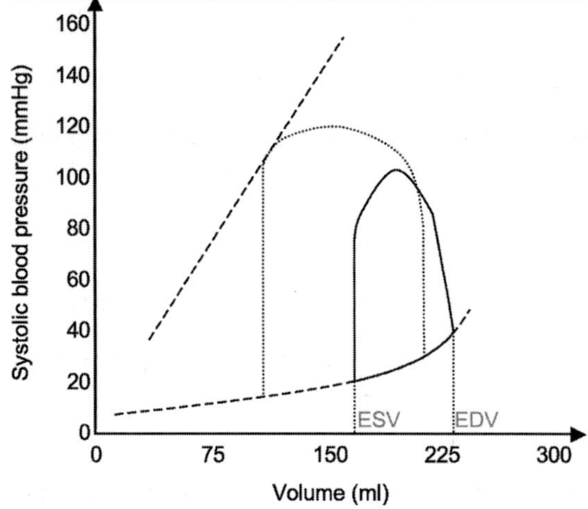

Draw and label the axes as shown. Note that the *x* axis should now contain higher values for volume as this plot will represent a distended failing ventricle. Plot a sample ESPVR and EDPVR as shown. Start by marking on the EDV at a higher volume than previously. Demonstrate that this point lies on the up-sloping segment of the EDPVR, causing a higher diastolic pressure than in the normal ventricle. Show that the curve is slurred during ventricular contraction rather than vertical, which suggests that there may be valvular incompetence. The peak pressure attainable by a failing ventricle may be lower as shown. The ESV should also be high, as ejection is compromised and the ventricle distended throughout its cycle. The EF is, therefore, reduced (30% in the above example) as is the stroke work.

Systemic and pulmonary vascular resistance

Systemic vascular resistance

The resistance to flow in the systemic circulation against which the left ventricle must contract (dyne.s.cm^{-5}).

Dyne

The force that will give a mass of 1 g an acceleration of 1 cm.s^{-2}.

The dyne is, therefore, numerically 1/100 000 of a newton and represents a tiny force.

Equation

Systemic blood pressure is a function of vascular resistance and cardiac output:

$$\text{SBP} = \text{CO} \times \text{SVR}$$

where SBP is systemic blood pressure, CO is cardiac output and SVR is systemic vascular resistance.

This relationship equates to the well-known relationship of Ohm's law:

$$V = IR$$

where SBP is equivalent to V (voltage), CO to I (current) and SVR to R (resistance).

To find resistance the equation must be rearranged as $R = V/I$ or

$$\text{SVR} = \frac{(\text{MAP} - \text{CVP})}{\text{CO}} \times 80$$

where MAP is mean arterial pressure, CVP is central venous pressure and 80 is a conversion factor. This can also be expressed as

$$\text{SVR} = \frac{(\text{MAP} - \text{RAP})}{\text{CO}} \times 80$$

where RAP is right atrial pressure.

A conversion factor of 80 is used to convert from the base units in the equation (mmHg and l.min^{-1}) to the commonly used units of the result (dyne.s.cm^{-5}). It is the pressure *difference* between input (CVP or RAP) and output (MAP) that is used in these equations rather than simply SBP. The SVR is usually 1000–1500 dyne.s.cm^{-5}.

Pulmonary vascular resistance

The resistance to flow in the pulmonary vasculature against which the right ventricle must contract (dyne.s.cm^{-5}):

$$PVR = \frac{(MPAP - LAP)}{CO} \times 80$$

where PVR is pulmonary vascular resistance, MPAP is mean pulmonary artery pressure and LAP is left atrial pressure.

The relationship for pulmonary vascular resistance is very non-linear owing to the effect of recruitment and distension of vessels in the pulmonary vascular bed in response to increased pulmonary blood flow. The PVR is usually around 10 times lower than the systemic vascular resistance, at 50–150 dyne.s.cm^{-5}.

The Valsalva manoeuvre

The patient is asked to forcibly exhale against a closed glottis for a period of 10 s. Blood pressure and heart rate are measured. Four phases occur during the manoeuvre. Phase 1 begins at the onset and is of short duration. Phase 2 continues until the end of the manoeuvre. Phase 3 begins as soon as the manoeuvre has finished and is of short duration. Phase 4 continues until restoration of normal parameters.

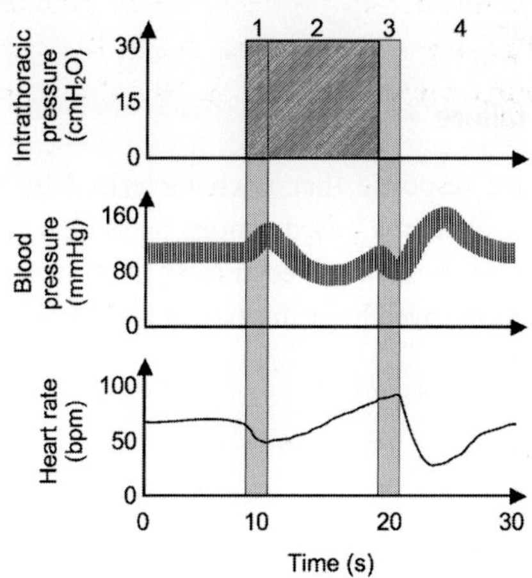

Draw and label all three axes. The uppermost trace shows the sustained rise in intrathoracic pressure during the 10 s of the manoeuvre. Mark the four phases on as vertical lines covering all three plot areas, so that your diagram can be drawn accurately.

Curves Draw normal heart rate and BP lines on the remaining two axes. Note that the BP line is thick so as to represent SBP at its upper border and DBP at its lower border.

Phase 1 During phase 1, the increased thoracoabdominal pressure transiently increases venous return, thereby raising BP and reflexly lowering heart rate.

Phase 2 During phase 2, the sustained rise in intrathoracic pressure reduces venous return VR and so BP falls until a compensatory tachycardia restores it.

Phase 3 The release of pressure in phase 3 creates a large empty venous reservoir, causing BP to fall. Show that the heart rate remains elevated.

Phase 4 The last phase shows how the raised heart rate then initially leads to a raised BP as venous return is restored. This is followed by a reflex bradycardia before both parameters eventually return to normal.

Uses

The Valsalva manoeuvre can be used to assess autonomic function or to terminate a supraventricular tachycardia.

Abnormal responses

Autonomic neuropathy/quadriplegia

There is an excessive drop in BP during phase 2 with no associated overshoot in phase 4. There is no bradycardia in phase 4. The response is thought to be caused by a diminished baroreceptor reflex and so the normal compensatory changes in heart rate do not occur.

Congestive cardiac failure

There is a square wave response that is characterized by a rise in BP during phase 2. This may be because the raised venous pressure seen with this condition enables venous return to be maintained during this phase. As with autonomic neuropathy, there is no BP overshoot in phase 4 and little change in heart rate.

Control of heart rate

The resting heart rate of 60–80 bpm results from dominant vagal tone. The intrinsic rate generated by the sinoatrial (SA) node is 110 bpm. Control of heart rate is, therefore, through the balance of parasympathetic and sympathetic activity via the vagus and cardioaccelerator (T1–T5) fibres, respectively.

Parasympathetic control

The pathway of parasympathetic control is shown below and acts via both the SA node and the atrioventricular (AV) node.

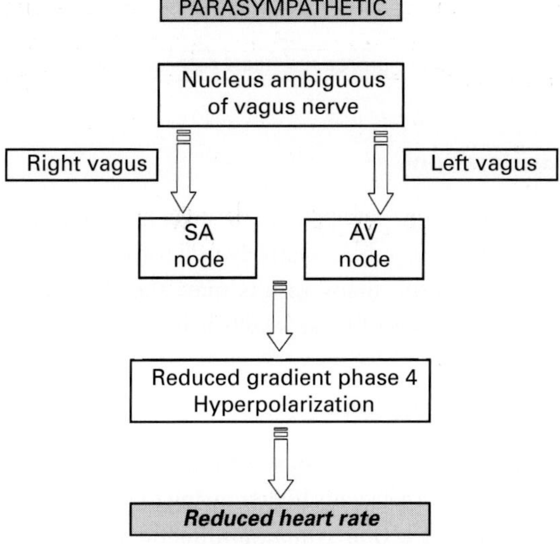

Sympathetic control

Sympathetic control is shown below.

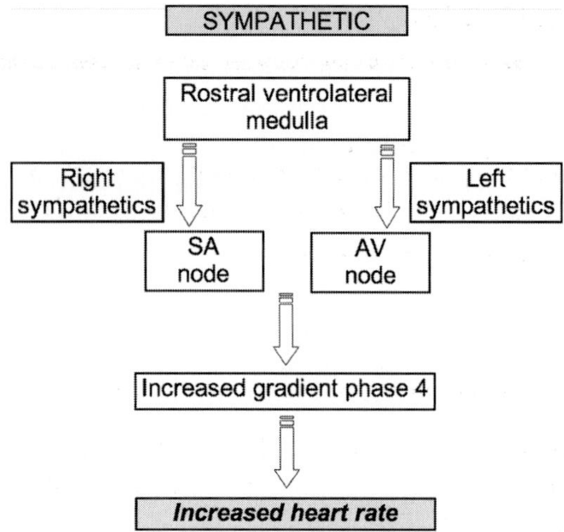

Paediatric considerations

In neonates and children the sympathetic system is relatively underdeveloped while the parasympathetic supply is relatively well formed. Despite a high resting heart rate in this population, many insults may, therefore, result in profound bradycardia. The most serious of these insults is hypoxia.

Post-transplant considerations

Following a heart transplant, both sympathetic and parasympathetic innervation is lost. The resting heart rate is usually higher owing to the loss of parasympathetic tone. Importantly, indirect acting sympathomimetic agents will have no effect. For example, ephedrine will be less effective as only its direct actions will alter heart rate. Atropine and glycopyrrolate will be ineffective and neostigmine may slow the heart rate and should be used with caution. Direct acting agents such as adrenaline (epinephrine) and isoprenaline will work and can be used with caution.

Acid–base balance

When considering the topic of acid–base balance, there are two key terms with which you should be familiar. These are pH and pK_a. Calculations of a patient's acid–base status will utilize these terms.

pH

The negative logarithm to the base 10 of the H^+ concentration.

Normal hydrogen ion concentration $[H^+]$ in the blood is 40 nmol.l^{-1}, giving a pH of 7.4. As pH is a logarithmic function, there must be a 10-fold change in $[H^+]$ for each unit change in pH.

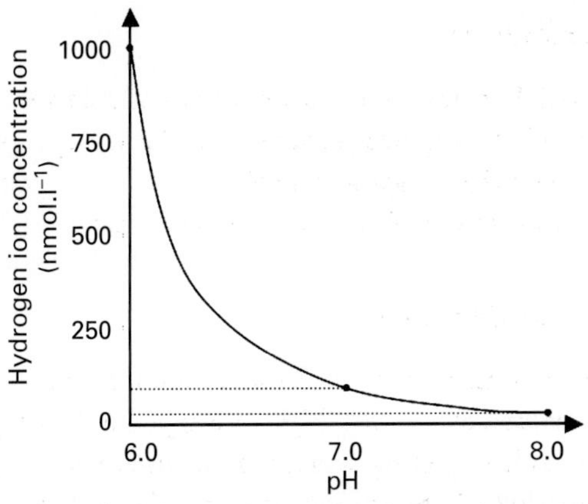

Draw and label the axes as shown. At a pH of 6, 7 and 8, $[H^+]$ is 1000, 100 and 10 nmol.l^{-1}, respectively. Plot these three points on the graph and join them with a smooth line to show the exponential relationship between the two variables.

pK_a

The negative logarithm of the dissociation constant.

or

The pH at which 50% of the drug molecules are ionized and 50% un-ionized.

The pK_a depends upon the molecular structure of the drug and is not related to whether the drug is an acid or a base.

Henderson–Hasselbach equation

The Henderson–Hasselbach equation allows the ratio of ionized:un-ionized compound to be found if the pH and pK_a are known. Consider carbonic acid (H_2CO_3) bicarbonate (HCO_3^-) buffer system

$$CO_2 + H_2O \leftrightarrow H_2CO_3 \leftrightarrow H^+ + HCO_3^-$$

Note that, by convention, the dissociation constant is labelled K_a ('a' for acid) as opposed to K_D, which is a more generic term. Although confusing, you should be aware that a difference in terminology exists.

The dissociation constant is given as

$$K_a = \frac{[H^+][HCO_3^-]}{[H_2CO_3]}$$

Taking logarithms gives

$$\log K_a = \log [H^+] + \log \frac{[HCO_3^-]}{[H_2CO_3]}$$

Subtract log [H$^+$] from both sides in order to move it to the left

$$\log K_a - \log [H^+] = \log \frac{[HCO_3^-]}{[H_2CO_3]}$$

Next do the same with log K_a in order to move it to the right

$$-\log [H^+] = -\log K_a + \log \frac{[HCO_3^-]}{[H_2CO_3]}$$

which can be written as

$$pH = pK_a + \log \frac{[HCO_3^-]}{[H_2CO_3]}$$

As H_2CO_3 is not routinely assayed, CO_2 may be used in its place. The blood [CO_2] is related to the $Pa\text{CO}_2$ by a factor of 0.23 mmol.l^{-1}.kPa^{-1} or 0.03 mmol.l^{-1}.mmHg^{-1}. The generic form of the equation states that, for an acid

$$pH = pK_a + \log \frac{[\text{ionized form}]}{[\text{un-ionized form}]}$$

and for a base

$$pH = pK_a + \log \frac{[\text{un-ionized form}]}{[\text{ionized form}]}$$

The Davenport diagram

The Davenport diagram shows the relationships between pH, $P\text{CO}_2$ and HCO_3^-. It can be used to explain the compensatory mechanisms that occur in acid–base balance. At first glance it appears complicated because of the number of lines but if it is drawn methodically it becomes easier to understand.

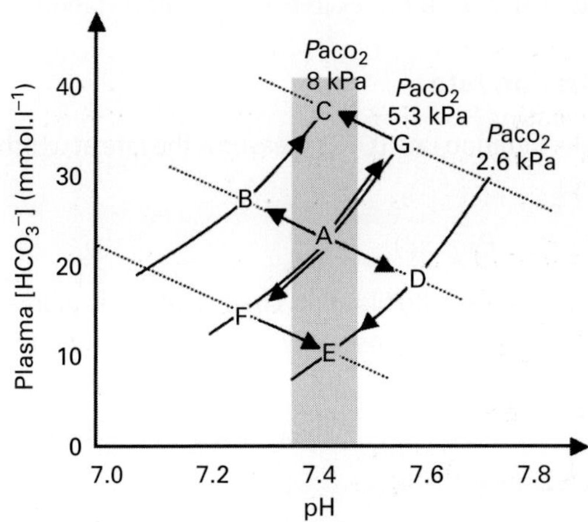

After drawing and labelling the axes, draw in the two sets of lines. The solid lines are lines of equal $P\text{aCO}_2$ and the dashed lines are the buffer lines. Normal plasma is represented by point A so make sure this point is accurately plotted. The shaded area represents the normal pH and points C and E should also lie in this area. The line BAD is the normal buffer line.

ABC Line AB represents a respiratory acidosis as the $P\text{aCO}_2$ has risen from 5.3 to 8 kPa. Compensation is shown by line BC, which demonstrates retention of HCO_3^-. The rise in HCO_3^- from 28 to 38 mmol.l^{-1} (*y* axis) returns the pH to the normal range.

AFE Line AF represents a metabolic acidosis as the HCO_3^- has fallen. Compensation occurs by hyperventilation and the $P\text{aCO}_2$ falls as shown by line FE.

ADE Line AD represents a respiratory alkalosis with the $P\text{aCO}_2$ falling to the 2.6 kPa line. Compensation is via loss of HCO_3^- to normalize pH, as shown by line DE.

AGC Line AG represents a metabolic alkalosis with a rise in HCO_3^- to 35 mmol.l^{-1}. Compensation occurs by hypoventilation along line GC.

Glomerular filtration rate

The balance of filtration at the glomerulus and reabsorption and secretion in the tubules allows the kidneys to maintain homeostasis of extracellular fluid, nutrients and acid–base balance and to excrete drugs and metabolic waste products.

Glomerular filtration rate

The glomerular filtration rate (GFR) measures the rate at which blood is filtered by the kidneys.

$$\mathrm{GFR} = K_\mathrm{f}(P_\mathrm{G} - P_\mathrm{B} - \pi_\mathrm{G})$$

where K_f is glomerular ultrafiltration coefficient, P_G is glomerular hydrostatic pressure, P_B is Bowman's capsule hydrostatic pressure and π_G is glomerular oncotic pressure.

or

$$\mathrm{GFR} = \mathrm{Clearance}$$

Clearance

The volume of plasma that is cleared of the substance per unit time ($\mathrm{ml.min^{-1}}$).

$$C_\mathrm{x} = \frac{U_\mathrm{x}V}{P_\mathrm{x}}$$

where C is clearance, U is urinary concentration, V is urine flow and P is plasma concentration.

Clearance is measured most accurately using inulin, which is freely filtered and not secreted, reabsorbed, metabolized or stored, but creatinine is a more practical surrogate.

Renal blood flow

Renal blood flow (RBF) is a function of renal plasma flow and the density of red blood cells.

$$\mathrm{RBF} = \mathrm{RPF}/(1 - \mathrm{Haematocrit})$$

Where RPF is renal plasma flow.

The RPF can be calculated using the same formula as the clearance formula but using a substance that is entirely excreted; *p*-aminohippuric acid is usually used.

$$\mathrm{RBF} = \frac{\mathrm{RPP}}{\mathrm{RVR}}$$

where RPP is renal perfusion pressure and RVR is renal vascular resistance.

This last equation follows the general rule of $V = I/R$.

Autoregulation and renal vascular resistance

Autoregulation of blood flow

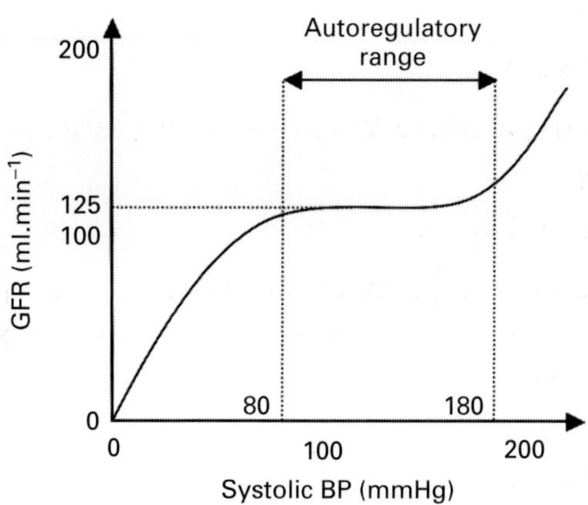

Draw and label the axes as shown. Your line should pass through the origin and rise as a straight line until it approaches 125 ml.min^{-1}. The flattening of the curve at this point demonstrates the beginning of the autoregulatory range. You should show that this range lies between 80 and 180 mmHg. At SBP values over 180 mmHg, your curve should again rise in proportion to the BP. Note that the line will eventually flatten out if systolic BP rises further, as a maximum GFR will be reached.

Renal vascular resistance

The balance of vascular tone between the afferent and efferent arterioles determines the GFR; therefore, changes in tone can increase or decrease GFR accordingly.

Afferent arteriole	Efferent arteriole	Result
Dilatation	**Constriction**	Increased GFR
Prostaglandins	Angiotensin II	
Kinins	Sympathetic stimulation	
Dopamine	Atrial natriuretic peptide	
Atrial natriuretic peptide		
Nitric oxide		

Afferent arteriole	Efferent arteriole	Result
Constriction	**Dilatation**	Reduced GFR
Angiotensin II	Angiotensin II blockade	
Sympathetic stimulation	Prostaglandins	
Endothelin		
Adenosine		
Vasopressin		
Prostaglandin blockade		

The loop of Henle

The function of the loop of Henle is to enable production of a concentrated urine. It does this by generating a hypertonic interstitium, which provides a gradient for water reabsorption from the collecting duct. This, in turn, occurs under the control of antidiuretic hormone (ADH). There are several important requirements without which this mechanism would not work. These include the differential permeabilities of the two limbs to water and solutes and the presence of a blood supply that does not dissipate the concentration gradients produced. This is a simplified description to convey the principles.

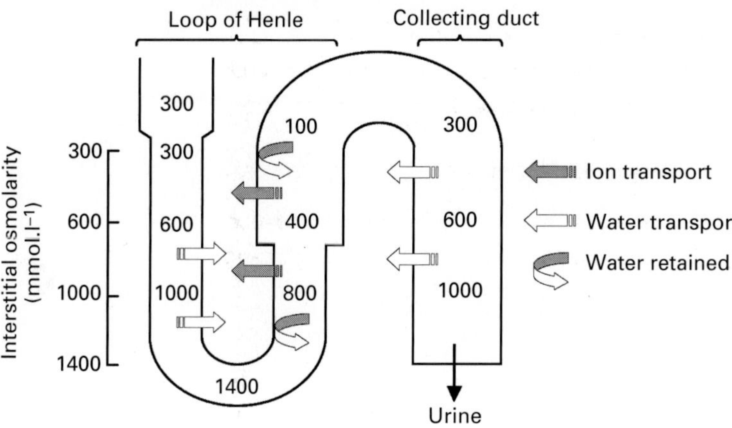

Start by drawing a schematic diagram of the tubule as shown above. Use the numerical values to explain what is happening to urine osmolarity in each region.

Descending limb Fluid entering is isotonic. Water moves out down a concentration gradient into the interstitium, concentrating the urine within the tubules.

Thin ascending limb Fluid entering is hypertonic. The limb is impermeable to water but ion transport does occur, which causes the urine osmolarity to fall.

Thick ascending limb This limb is also impermeable to water. It contains ion pumps to pump electrolytes actively into the interstitium. The main pump is the $Na^+/2Cl^-/K^+$ co-transporter. Fluid leaving this limb is, therefore, hypotonic and passes into the distal convoluted tubule.

Collecting duct The duct has selective permeability to water, which is controlled by ADH. In the presence of ADH, water moves into the interstitium down the concentration gradient generated by the loop of Henle.

Glucose handling

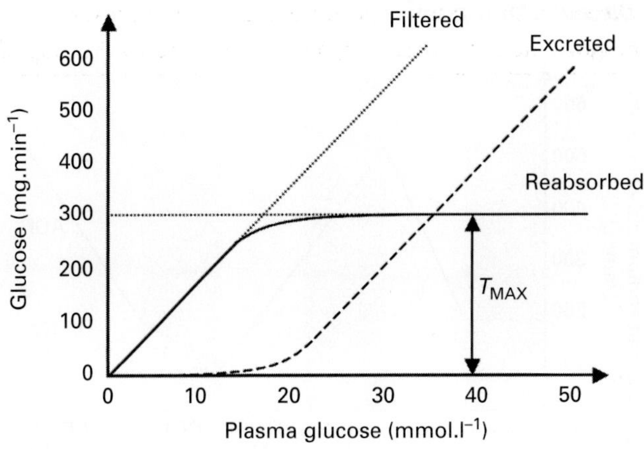

Filtered After drawing and labelling the axes, draw a line passing through origin, rising at an angle of approximately 45°. This demonstrates that the amount of glucose filtered by the kidney is directly proportional to the plasma glucose concentration.

Reabsorbed This line also passes through the origin. It matches the 'filtered' line until 11 mmol.l^{-1} and then starts to flatten out as it approaches maximal tubular reabsorption (T_{MAX}). Demonstrate that this value is 300 mg.min^{-1} on the *y* axis.

Excreted Glucose can only appear in the urine when the two lines drawn so far begin to separate so that less is reabsorbed than is filtered. This happens at 11 mmol.l^{-1} plasma glucose concentration. The line then rises parallel to the 'filtered' line as plasma glucose continues to rise.

Sodium handling

Sodium concentration graph

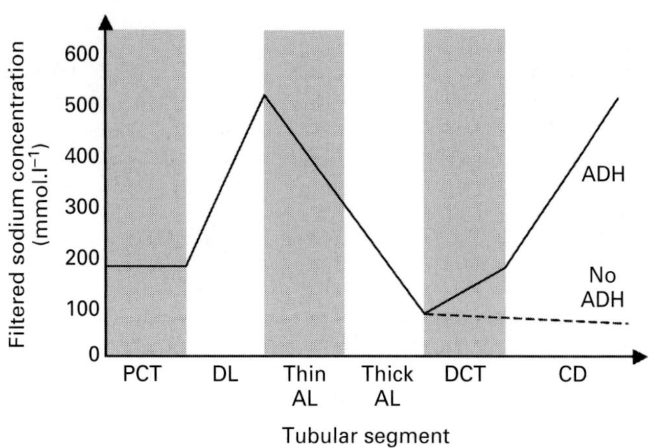

PCT is proximal convoluted tubule, DL is descending limb of the loop of Henle, Thin AL is thin ascending limb of the loop of Henle, Thick AL is thick ascending limb of the loop of Henle, DCT is distal convoluted tubule and CD is collecting duct. (This figure is reproduced with permission from *Fundamental Principles and Practice of Anaesthesia*, P. Hutton, G. Cooper, F. James and J. Butterworth. Martin-Dunitz 2002 pp. 487, illustration no. 25.16.)

The graph shows how the concentration of Na^+ in the filtrate changes as it passes along the tubule. An important point to demonstrate is how much of an effect ADH has on the final urinary $[Na^+]$. Draw and label the axes as shown. The initial concentration should be just below 200 mmol.l^{-1}. The loop of Henle is the site of the countercurrent exchange mechanism so should result in a highly concentrated filtrate at its tip, 500–600 mol.l^{-1} is usual. By the end of the thick ascending limb, you should demonstrate that the urine is now hypotonic with a low $[Na^+]$ of approximately 100 mmol.l^{-1}. The presence of maximal ADH will act on the distal convoluted tubule and collecting duct to retain water and deliver a highly concentrated urine with a high $[Na^+]$ of approximately 600 mmol.l^{-1}. Conversely, show that in the absence of ADH the urinary $[Na^+]$ may be as low as 80–100 mmol.l^{-1}.

Potassium handling

Potassium concentration graph

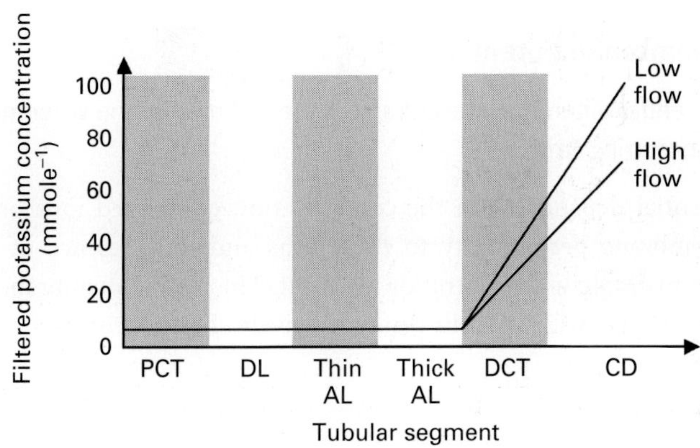

PCT is proximal convoluted tubule, DL is descending limb of the loop of Henle, Thin AL is thin ascending limb of the loop of Henle, Thick AL is thick ascending limb of the loop of Henle, DCT is distal convoluted tubule and CD is collecting duct. (Reproduced with permission from *Fundamental Principles and Practice of Anaesthesia*, P. Hutton, G. Cooper, F. James and J. Butterworth. Martin-Dunitz 2002 pp. 488, illustration no. 25.17.)

The graph shows how the filtrate $[K^+]$ changes as it passes along the tubule. Draw and label the axes as shown. The curve is easier to remember as it stays essentially horizontal at a concentration of approximately 5–10 mmol.l^{-1} until the distal convoluted tubule. Potassium is secreted here along electrochemical gradients, which makes it unusual. You should demonstrate that at low urinary flow rates, tubular $[K^+]$ is higher at approximately 100 mmol.l^{-1} and so less K^+ is excreted as the concentration gradient is reduced. Conversely, at higher urinary flow rates (as are seen with diuretic usage) the $[K^+]$ may only be 70 mmol.l^{-1} and so secretion is enhanced. In this way, K^+ loss from the body may actually be greater when the $[K^+]$ of the urine is lower, as total loss equals urine flow multiplied by concentration.

Action potentials

Resting membrane potential

The potential difference present across the cell membrane when no stimulation is occurring (mV).

The potential depends upon the concentration of charged ions present, the relative membrane permeability to those ions and the presence of any ionic pumps that maintain a concentration gradient. The resting membrane potential is – 60 to – 90 mV, with the cells being negatively charged inside.

Action potential

The spontaneous depolarization of an excitable cell in response to a stimulus.

Gibbs–Donnan effect

The differential separation of charged ions across a semipermeable membrane.

The movement of solute across a semipermeable membrane depends upon the chemical concentration gradient and the electrical gradient. Movement occurs down the concentration gradient until a significant opposing electrical potential has developed. This prevents further movement of ions and the Gibbs–Donnan equilibrium is reached. This is electrochemical equilibrium and the potential difference across the cell is the equilibrium potential. It can be calculated using the Nernst equation.

The Nernst equation

$$E = \frac{RT}{zF} \cdot \ln \frac{[C_o]}{[C_i]}$$

where E is the equilibrium potential, R is the universal gas constant, T is absolute temperature, z is valency and F is Faraday's constant.

The values for Cl^-, Na^+ and K^+ are − 70, + 60 and − 90 mV, respectively. Note that the equation only gives an equilibrium for individual ions. If more than one ion is involved in the formation of a membrane potential, a different equation must be used, as shown below.

Goldman constant field equation

$$E = \frac{RT}{F} \cdot \ln \frac{([Na^+]_o.P_{Na^+} + [K^+]_o.P_{K^+} + [Cl^-]_o.P_{Cl^-})}{([Na^+]_i.P_{Na^+} + [K^+]_i.P_{K^+} + [Cl^-]_i.P_{Cl^-})}$$

where E is membrane potential, R is the universal gas constant, T is absolute temperature, F is Faraday's constant, $[X]_o$ is the concentration of given ion outside the cell, $[X]_i$ is the concentration of given ion inside cell and P_X is the permeability of given ion.

Action potentials

You will be expected to have an understanding of action potentials in nerves, cardiac pacemaker cells and cardiac conduction pathways.

Absolute refractory period

The period of time following the initiation of an action potential when no stimulus will elicit a further response (ms).

It usually lasts until repolarization is one third complete and corresponds to the increased Na^+ conductance that occurs during this time.

Relative refractory period

The period of time following the initiation of an action potential when a larger than normal stimulus may result in a response (ms).

This is the time from the absolute refractory period until the cell's membrane potential is less than the threshold potential. It corresponds to the period of increased K^+ conductance.

Threshold potential

The membrane potential that must be achieved for an action potential to be propagated (mV).

Nerve action potential

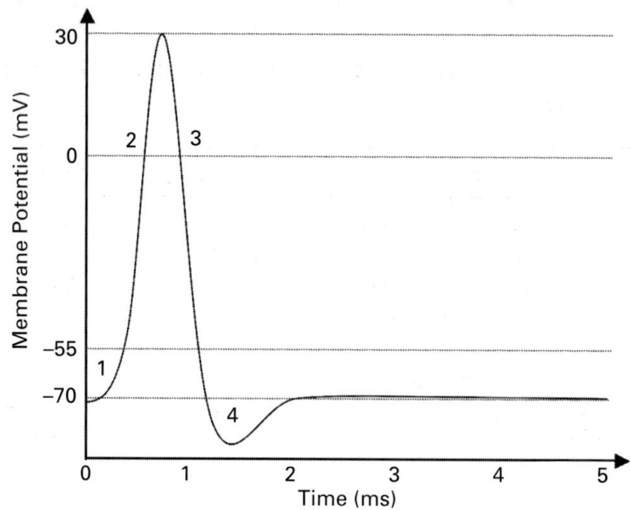

Draw and label the axes as shown.

Phase 1 The curve should cross the *y* axis at approximately $-70\,\text{mV}$ and should be shown to rapidly rise towards the threshold potential of $-55\,\text{mV}$.

Phase 2 This portion of the curve demonstrates the rapid rise in membrane potential to a peak of $+30\,\text{mV}$ as voltage-gated Na^+ channels allow rapid Na^+ entry into the cell.

Phase 3 This phase shows rapid repolarization as Na^+ channels close and K^+ channels open, allowing K^+ efflux. The slope of the downward curve is almost as steep as that seen in phase 2.

Phase 4 Show that the membrane potential 'overshoots' in a process known as hyperpolarization as the Na^+/K^+ pump lags behind in restoring the normal ion balance.

Cardiac action potential

For cardiac action potentials and pacemaker potentials see Section 7.

Types of neurone

You may be asked about different types of nerve fibre and their function. The table is complicated but remember that the largest fibres conduct at the fastest speeds. If you can remember some of the approximate values given below it will help to polish your answer.

Fibre type	Function	Diameter (μm)	Conduction ($m.s^{-1}$)
Aα	Proprioception, motor	10–20	100
Aβ	Touch, pressure	5–10	50
Aγ	Muscle spindle motor	2–5	25
Aδ	Pain, temperature, touch	2–5	25
B (autonomic)	Preganglionic	3	10
C	Pain, temperature	1	1
C (sympathetic)	Postganglionic	1	1

Velocity calculations

For myelinated nerves

$$V \propto d$$

where V is the velocity of transmission and d is the diameter of the neurone.

For unmyelinated nerves

$$V \propto \sqrt{d}$$

Muscle structure and function

Neuromuscular junction

You may be questioned on the structure and function of the neuromuscular junction and could be expected to illustrate your answer with a diagram. A well-drawn diagram will make your answer clearer.

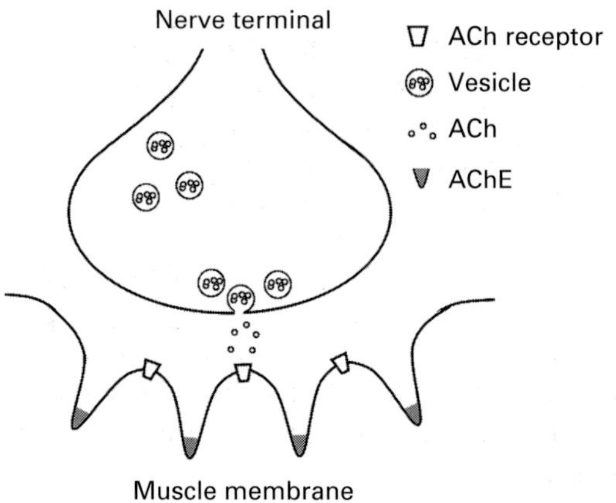

The diagram shows the synaptic cleft, which is found at the junction of the nerve terminal and the muscle membrane.

Vesicle You should demonstrate that there are two stores of acetylcholine (ACh), one deep in the nerve terminal and one clustered beneath the surface opposite the ACh receptors in the so-called 'active zones'. The deep stores serve as a reserve of ACh while those in the active zones are required for immediate release of ACh into the synaptic cleft.

ACh receptor These are located on the peaks of the junctional folds of the muscle membrane as shown. They are also found presynaptically on the nerve terminal, where, once activated, they promote migration of ACh vesicles from deep to superficial stores.

Acetylcholinesterase (AChE) This enzyme is found in the troughs of the junctional folds of the muscle membrane and is responsible for metabolizing ACh within the synaptic cleft.

Sarcomere

The contractile unit of the myocyte.

You may be asked to draw a diagram of the sarcomere. It is made up of actin and myosin filaments, as shown below. The thick myosin filaments contain many cross-bridges, which, when activated, bind to the thin actin filaments. Tropomyosin molecules (containing troponin) run alongside the actin filaments and play an important role in excitation–contraction coupling.

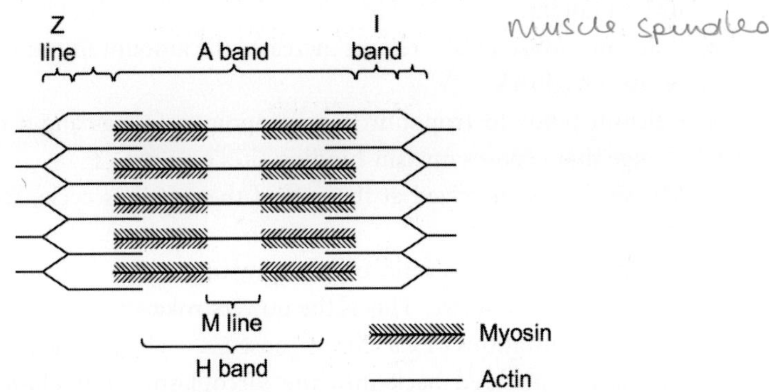

The diagram should be drawn carefully so that the actin and myosin filaments are shown to overlap while ensuring that enough space is left between them to identify the various lines and bands.

Z line The junction between neighbouring actin filaments that forms the border between sarcomeres. It has a Z-shaped appearance on the diagram.

M line The 'middle' zone of the sarcomere, formed from the junction between neighbouring myosin filaments. There are no cross-bridges in this region.

A band This band spans the length of the myosin filament although it is confusingly given the letter A.

I band This band represents the portion of actin filaments that are not overlapped by myosin. It comes 'in between' the Z line and the A band.

H band This band represents the portion of the myosin filaments that are not overlapped by actin.

Excitation–contraction coupling

The series of physiological events that link the depolarization of the muscle membrane to contraction of the muscle fibre.

This is a complicated chain of events that can easily cause confusion in the examination setting. The list below gives a summary of the salient points.

1. The action potential is conducted into muscle fibre by T-tubules.
2. Depolarization of the T-tubules results in calcium release from the sarcoplasmic reticulum.
3. Calcium-induced Ca^{2+} release increases the amount of intracellular Ca^{2+} by positive feedback.
4. Calcium binds to troponin C on tropomyosin, causing a conformational change that exposes myosin-binding sites on actin.
5. Myosin heads energized at the end of the previous cycle, can now bind to actin.
6. Binding of myosin to actin triggers pivoting of the myosin head and shortening of the sarcomere. This is the powerstroke.
7. High concentrations of Ca^{2+} now cause Ca^{2+} channel closure.
8. Calcium is pumped back into the sarcoplasmic reticulum. This requires adenosine triphosphate (ATP).
9. ATP binds to the myosin cross-bridges, leading to release of the bond between actin and myosin.
10. The ATP is hydrolysed, energizing the myosin ready for the next contraction.
11. The muscle relaxes.
12. The decreased $[Ca^{2+}]$ causes tropomyosin to resume its previous configuration, blocking the myosin-binding site.

Muscle reflexes

There is only one monosynaptic reflex known to exist in humans – the stretch reflex. For this reason, it is commonly examined and an overview of its components and their functions is given below.

The stretch reflex

A monosynaptic reflex responsible for the control of posture.

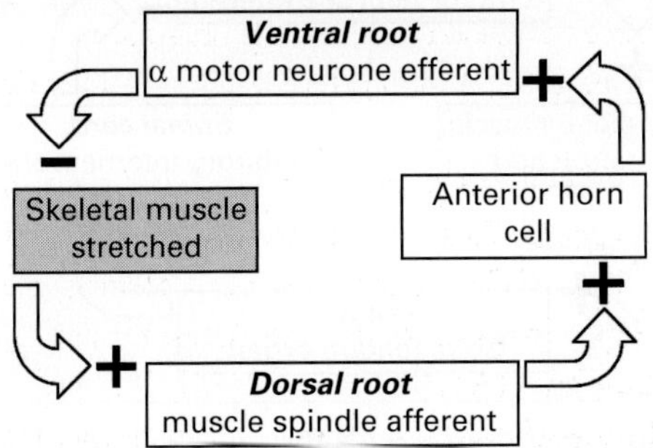

Stretching of the muscle is sensed in the muscle spindle and leads to firing in muscle spindle afferent. These nerves travel via the dorsal root and synapse in the anterior horn of the spinal cord directly with the motor neurone to that muscle. They stimulate firing of the motor neurones, which causes contraction of the muscle that has just been stretched. The muscle spindle afferent also synapses with inhibitory interneurons, which inhibit the antagonistic muscles. This is called reciprocal innervation.

Muscle spindles

Stretch transducers encapsulated in the muscle fibre responsible for maintenance of a constant muscle length despite changes in the load.

Muscle spindles are composed of nuclear bag (dynamic) and chain (static) fibres known as intrafusal fibres and these are innervated by γ motor neurones. Extrafusal fibres make up the muscle bulk and are innervated by α motor neurones. Stimulation of the muscle spindle leads to increased skeletal muscle contraction, which opposes the initial stretch and maintains the length of the fibre. This feedback loop oscillates at 10 Hz, which is the frequency of a physiological tremor.

In the same way that muscle spindles are responsible for the maintenance of muscle length, Golgi tendon organs are responsible for maintenance of muscle tension.

Golgi tendon organs

These are found in muscle tendons and monitor the tension in the muscle. Their function is to limit the tension that is generated in the muscle.

Tension is the force that is being opposed by the muscle and is a different concept to stretch. The reflex can be summarized as below.

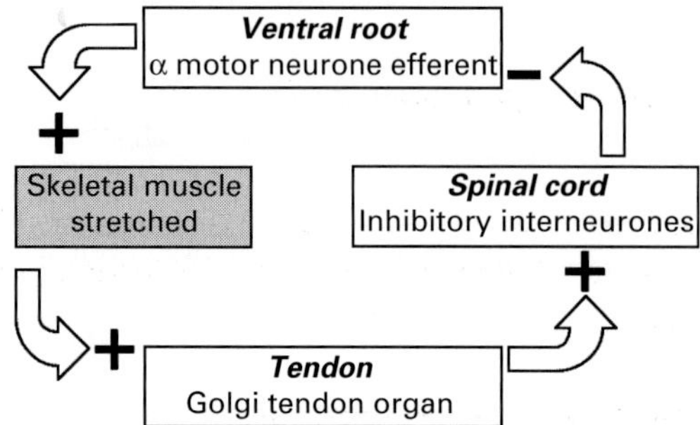

Golgi tendon organs are in series with the muscle fibres. They are stimulated by an increase in tension in the muscle, which may be passive owing to muscle stretch or active owing to muscle contraction. Stimulation results in increased firing in afferent nerve fibres, which causes inhibition of the muscle in question, increasing muscle stretch and, therefore, regulating muscle tension. The antagonistic muscle is simultaneously stimulated to contract.

All these muscle reflexes are under the control of descending motor pathways and are integrated in the spinal cord.

The Monro–Kelly doctrine

The skull is a rigid container of constant volume. The Monro–Kelly doctrine states that any increase in the volume of one of its contents must be compensated for by a reduction in volume of another if a rise in intracranial pressure (ICP) is to be avoided.

This volume of the skull comprises three compartments:

- brain (85%)
- cerebrospinal fluid (CSF) (10%)
- blood (5%).

Compensation for a raised ICP normally occurs in three stages. Initially there is a reduction in venous blood volume followed by a reduction in CSF volume and finally arterial blood volume.

Intracranial volume–pressure relationship

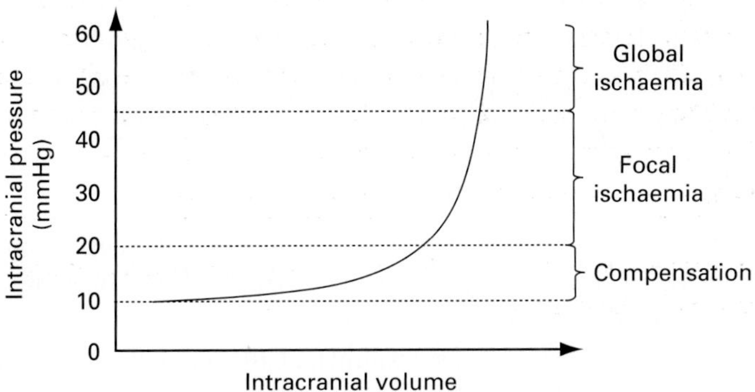

> Draw and label the axes as shown. Note that the *x* axis is usually drawn without any numerical markers. Normal intracranial volume is assumed to be at the left side of the curve and should be in keeping with an ICP of 5–10 mmHg. Draw a curve similar in shape to a positive tear-away exponential. Demonstrate on your curve that compensation for a rise in the volume of one intracranial component maintains the ICP < 20 mmHg. However, when these limited compensatory mechanisms are exhausted, ICP rises rapidly, causing focal ischaemia (ICP 20–45 mmHg) followed by global ischaemia (ICP > 45 mmHg).

Intracranial pressure relationships

Autoregulation

The ability of an organ to regulate its blood flow despite changes in its perfusion pressure.

Autoregulation of cerebral blood flow

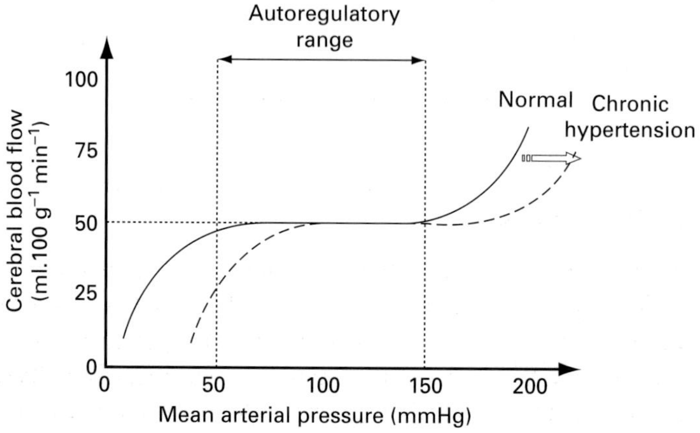

Draw and label the axes as shown. Mark the two key points on the x axis (50 and 150 mmHg). Between these points, mark a horizontal line at a y value of 50 ml.100g^{-1}.min^{-1}. Label this segment the 'autoregulatory range'. Above this range, cerebral blood flow (CBF) will increase as mean arterial pressure (MAP) increases. There will, however, be a maximum flow at some MAP where no further increase is possible. Below 50 mmHg, CBF falls with MAP; however, the line does not pass through the origin as neither MAP nor flow can be zero in live patients. Demonstrate the response to chronic hypertension by drawing an identical curve displaced to the right to show how the autoregulatory range 'resets' itself under these conditions.

Cerebral perfusion pressure

$$CPP = MAP - (ICP + CVP)$$

where CPP is cerebral perfusion pressure and CVP is central venous pressure.

Often, CVP is left out of this equation as it is normally negligible. In order to maintain cerebral perfusion when ICP is raised, the MAP must also be elevated.

Effects of Pa_{CO_2} on cerebral blood flow

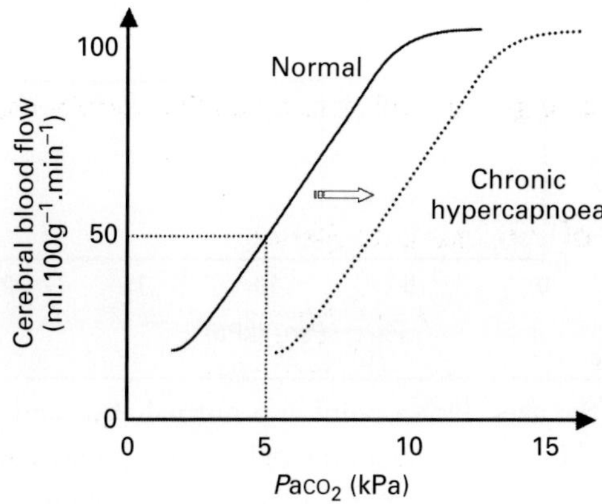

Draw and label the axes.

Normal Mark a point at the intersection of a normal Pa_{CO_2} and cerebral blood flow as shown. As CBF will approximately double with a doubling of the Pa_{CO_2} extend a line from this point up to a Pa_{CO_2} of around 10 kPa. At the extremes of Pa_{CO_2} there arise minimum and maximum flows that depend on maximal and minimal vasodilatation, respectively. The line should, therefore, become horizontal as shown at these extremes.

Chronic hypercapnoea The curve is identical but shifted to the right of the normal curve as buffering acts to reset the autoregulatory range.

Effects of Pa_{O_2} on cerebral blood flow

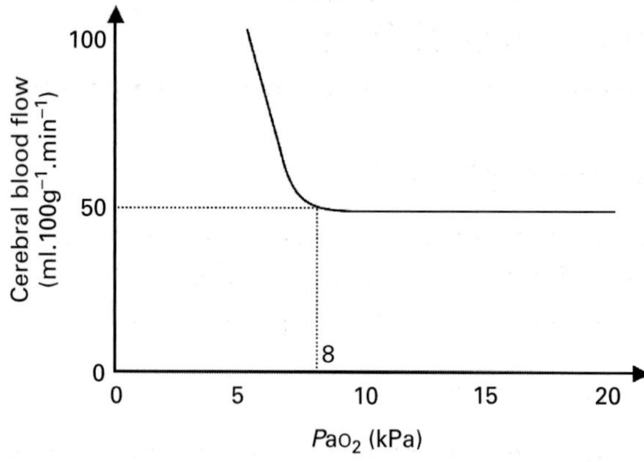

Draw and label the axes. Plot a point at a normal Pa_{O_2} and CBF as shown. Draw a horizontal line extending to the right of this point. This demonstrates that for values >8 kPa on the *x* axis, CBF remains constant. Below this point, hypoxia causes cerebral vasodilatation and CBF rises rapidly. At flow rates >100 ml.100g^{-1}.min^{-1}, maximal blood flow will be attained and the curve will tail off. Remember that the vasodilatory effect of hypoxia will override any other reflexes to ensure maximal oxygenation of the brain tissue.

Formation and circulation of cerebrospinal fluid

Formation of cerebrospinal fluid

The choroid plexus in the ventricles of the brain produce CSF at a constant rate of 500 $ml.day^{-1}$ or 0.35 $ml.min^{-1}$. The total volume of CSF is around 150 ml in the average adult. The rate of reabsorption of CSF is proportional to its outflow pressure.

Circulation of cerebrospinal fluid

An understanding of this well-documented circulatory route for CSF will be expected in the examinations.

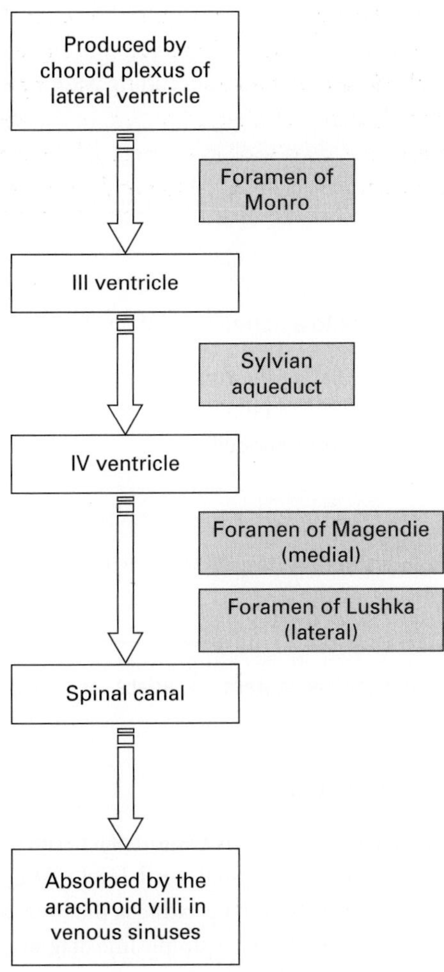

Pain

Pain is an unpleasant sensory and/or emotional experience associated with actual or potential tissue damage.

Chronic pain

Pain that persists after removal of the stimulus and beyond the normal recovery period.

Some believe that pain should be present for at least 3 months in order to be 'chronic' although most examiners should accept the definition above.

Nociception

The sensation of the noxious stimulus occurring within the brain.

Allodynia

A painful response to a normally painless stimulus.

Hyperalgesia

An exaggerated response to a normally painful stimulus.

Primary hyperalgesia occurs within the zone of injury and is caused by changes at the injury site itself. Secondary hyperalgesia occurs around the zone of injury and results from neuroplasticity and remodelling.

Hyperpathia

Pain in response to a stimulus despite sensory impairment.

Plasticity

The ability of the nervous system to adapt or change according to its environment.

The gate control theory of pain

Melzack and Wall theorized that the transmission of a peripheral painful stimulus to the CNS occurs via a 'gate' at spinal cord level. This gate comprises an inhibitory interneurone in the substantia gelatinosa that may be either stimulated or inhibited by different afferent inputs. A simple line diagram can be useful when explaining the mechanism to avoid confusion.

Neuronal connections

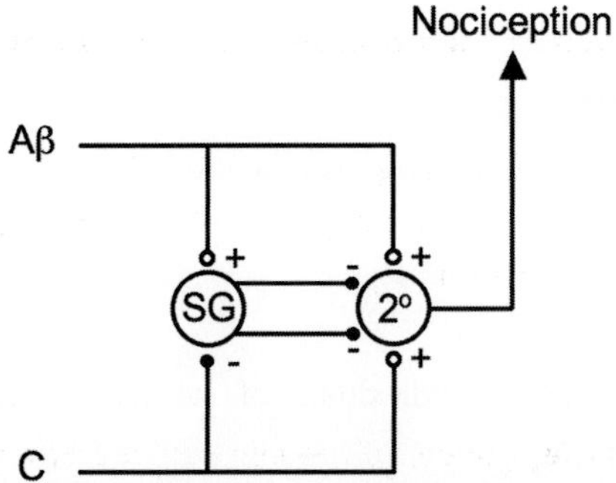

The Aβ fibres are examples of afferents that stimulate inhibitory interneurones (in the substantia gelatinosa (SG)) and, therefore, prevent nociceptive transmission to the CNS. The C fibres are examples of afferents that inhibit inhibitory interneurones and, therefore, enhance nociceptive transmission. Note that both types of fibre stimulate the second-order neurone (2°) directly but it is the interneurone that modifies the transmission.

Pain pathway

The diagram below shows the pathway of pain transmission from the peripheral nerves to the cerebral cortex. There are three levels of neuronal involvement and the signals may be modulated at two points during their course to the cerebral cortex. Descending inhibitory pathways arise in the midbrain and pass to the dorsal horn as shown. Multiple different neurotransmitters are involved in the pathway and include gamma-aminobutyric acid (GABA), *N*-methyl-D-aspartate (NMDA), noradrenaline and opioids.

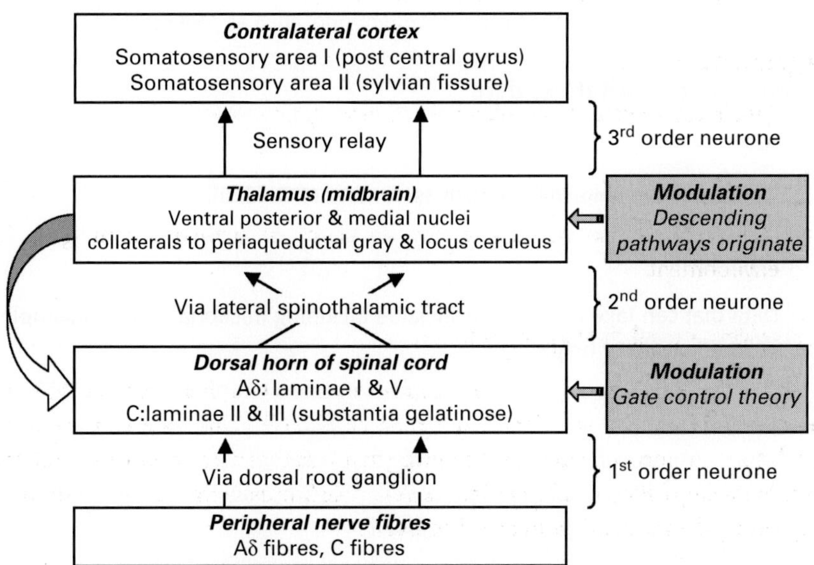

Data types

Population

The entire number of individuals of which the sample aims to be representative.

Sample

A group taken from the wider population. A sample aims to be representative of the population from which it is taken.

As samples are smaller, they are easier to collect and to analyse statistically. However, as they do not contain all of the values in the population, they can misrepresent it. Statistical analysis is often used to decide whether samples of data come from the same or from different populations. Populations are described by parameters and samples by statistics.

Categorical (qualitative) data

Nominal

Data that have no numerically significant order, such as blood groups.

Ordinal

Data that have an implicit order of magnitude, such as ASA score.

Numerical (quantitative) data

Discrete

Data that have finite values, such as number of children.

Continuous

Data that can take any numerical value including fractional values. Examples include weight or height.

Ratio

Any data series that has zero as its baseline value, for example blood pressure or the Kelvin temperature scale.

Interval

Any data series that includes zero as a point on a larger scale, for example the centigrade temperature scale.

There is a hierarchy of usefulness of data, according to how well it can be statistically manipulated. The accepted order is continuous data > ordinal data > nominal data.

Indices of central tendency and variability

Describing data

Once data have been collected, the values will be distributed around a central point or points. Various terms are used to describe both the measure of central tendency and the spread of data points around it.

Measures of central tendency

Mean

> The average value: the sum of the data values divided by the number of data points. Denoted by the symbol $\bar{x}$ when describing a sample mean and μ when describing a population mean.

The mean is always used when describing the normal distribution and, therefore, it is the most important measure with regards to the examination.

Median

> The middle value of a data series, having 50% of the data points above it and 50% below.

If there are an even number of data points, the median value is assumed to be the average of the middle two values.

Mode

> The most frequently occurring value in a set of data points.

The data can be plotted on a graph to demonstrate the distribution of the values. The individual values are plotted on the x axis with the frequency with which they occur on the y axis.

Measures of spread

Variance

> A measure of the spread of data around a central point. Described by the following equation.

$$\text{Var} = \frac{\Sigma(\bar{x} - x)^2}{n - 1}$$

Standard deviation

A measure of the spread of data around a central point. Described by the following equation (σ for population, SD for sample):

$$SD = \sqrt{\frac{\Sigma(\bar{x} - x)^2}{n - 1}}$$

Begin by finding the mean value ($\bar{x}$) of the distribution and then subtract each data point from it to find the difference between the values

$$\bar{x} - x$$

Square the results to ensure that all values are positive numbers:

$$(\bar{x} - x)^2$$

Sum the results:

$$\Sigma(\bar{x} - x)^2$$

Next divide the result by the number of observations (minus 1 for statistical reasons) to give the mean spread or variance

$$\frac{\Sigma(\bar{x} - x)^2}{n - 1}$$

The units for variance are, therefore, squared, which can cause difficulties. If the observations are measuring time for instance, the variance may be given in seconds squared (s^2), which is meaningless. The square root of the variance is, therefore, used to return to the original units. This is the SD.

$$SD = \sqrt{\frac{\Sigma(\bar{x} - x)^2}{n - 1}}$$

The spread of data is often described by quoting the percentage of the sample or population that will fall within a certain range. For the normal distribution, 1SD either side of the mean will contain 68% of all data points, 1.96SD 95%, 2SD 95.7% and 3SD 99.7%.

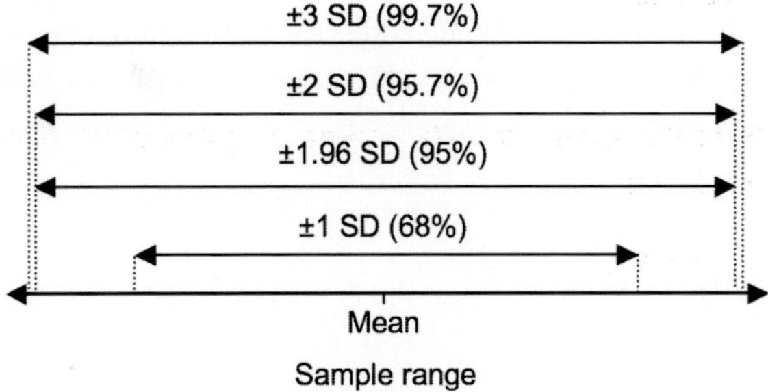

Standard error of the mean

The standard deviation of a group of sample means taken from the same population (SEM):

$$\text{SEM} = \sigma/\sqrt{(n-1)}$$

where σ is the SD of the population and n is the number in the samples.

In practice, the population SD is unlikely to be known and so the sample SD is used instead, giving

$$\text{SEM} = \text{SD}/\sqrt{(n-1)}$$

In the same way as the SD is used as a measure of spread around a mean, the SEM is used as a measure of the spread of a group of sample means around the true population mean. It is used to predict how closely the sample mean reflects the population mean.

As the sample size increases, SEM becomes smaller. For this reason, the SEM is sometimes quoted in study results rather than the SD in order to make the data look better.

Degrees of freedom

Statistics frequently involve calculations of the mean of a sample. In order to be able to calculate a mean, there must be at least two values present. For this reason, when describing sample size, the term $n-1$ is often used instead of the actual number. One of the sample points *must* be present in order that each of the other points can be used in the mean calculation. In other words, the size of the freely chosen sample must always be one less than are actually present.

For large sample sizes, the correction factor makes no difference to the calculation, but for small sample sizes it can be quite important. It is, therefore, best always to describe the sample size in this way.

Confidence intervals

The range of values that will contain the true population mean with a stated percentage confidence. Used in parametric tests.

A 95% confidence interval is ±1.96SD and is the most frequently quoted. There is a 95% certainty that this range of values around the mean will contain the population mean.

Quartile

Any one of the three values that divide a given range of data into four equal parts.

In order to tear a piece of paper into four equally wide strips, three tears must be made. One to tear the original paper in half and the other two to tear those halves in half again. A quartile is the mathematical equivalent of this to a range of ordered data. You should realize that the middle quartile (Q_2) is, in effect, the median for the range. Similarly, the first quartile (Q_1) is effectively the median of the lower half of the dataset and the third quartile (Q_3) the median of the upper half. In the same way as for the median calculation, a quartile should be represented as the mean of two data points if it lies between them.

Interquartile range

The range of values that lie between the first and third quartiles and, therefore, represent 50% of the data points. Used in non-parametric tests.

Calculating quartiles and using the interquartile range is useful in order to negate the effect of extreme values in a dataset, which tend to create a less stable statistic.

Types of distribution

The normal distribution

A bell-shaped distribution in which the mean, median and mode all have the same value, with defined SD distribution as above.

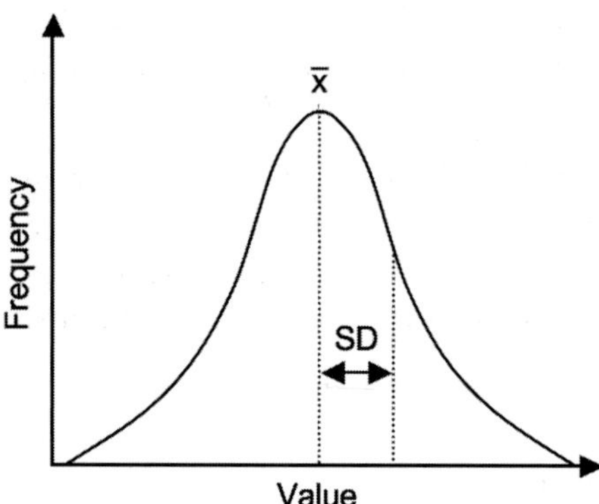

The curve is symmetrical around the mean, which is numerically identical to the median and mode. The SD should be indicated; 1SD lies approximately one third of the way between $\bar{x}$ and the end of the curve.

Positively skewed distribution

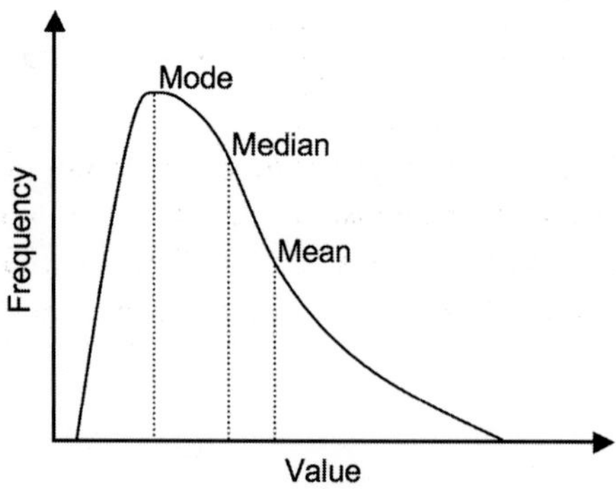

The curve is asymmetrical with a longer tail stretching off towards the more positive values. The mean, median and mode are now separated so that $\bar{x}$ is nearest the tail of the curve; the mode is at the peak frequency and the median is in between the two. This type of distribution can sometimes be made normal by logarithmic transformation of the data.

Negatively skewed distribution

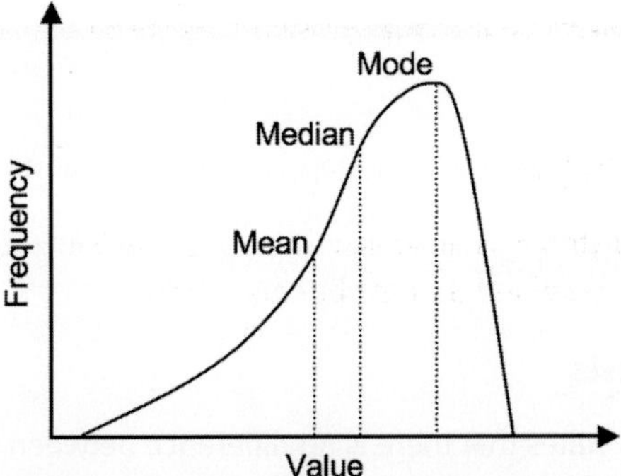

The curve is asymmetrical with a longer tail stretching off towards the more negative values. The mean, median and mode are now separated in the other direction, with $\bar{x}$ remaining closest to the tail. This type of distribution can sometimes be made normal by performing a power transformation (squaring or cubing the data).

Bimodal distribution

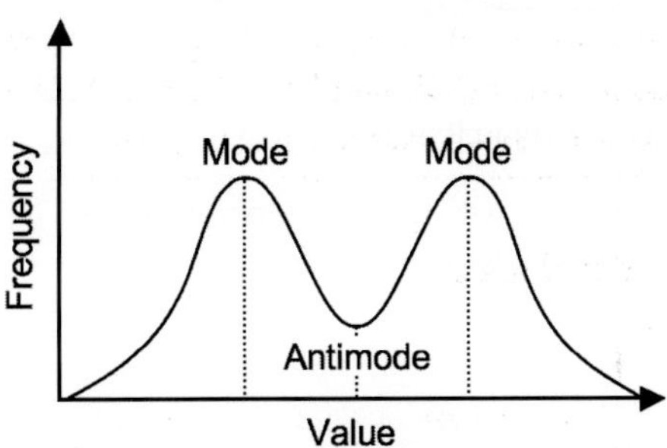

The curve need not be symmetrical nor have two modes of exactly the same height but the above curve demonstrates the principle well. The low point between the modes is known as the antimode. This curve could represent the heights of the population, with one mode for men and one for women.

Methods of data analysis

When performing a study, the first step is to pose a question. The question is formulated as a hypothesis that must be proved or disproved. This question is known as the null hypothesis.

The null hypothesis

The hypothesis states that there is no difference between the sample groups; that is, they both are from the same population (H_0).

The study then examines whether this is true. The amount of data needed to prove a difference between the samples depends on the size of the difference that is to be detected. Enough data must be collected to minimize the risk of a false-positive or false-negative result. This is determined by a power calculation.

Power

The ability of a statistical test to reveal a difference of a certain magnitude (%):

$$1 - \beta$$

where β is the β error (type II error).

Acceptable power is 80–90%, which equates to a β value of 10–20%. In effect, this means a 10–20% chance of a false-negative result.

The *p* value

The likelihood of the observed value being a result of chance alone.

Conventionally a p (probability) value of < 0.05 is taken to mean statistical significance. This means that if $p = 0.05$ then the observed difference could occur by chance on 1 in 20 (5%) of occasions. In effect, this means a 5% chance of a false-positive result.

Number needed to treat

The number of patients that have to be treated to prevent one outcome event occurring.

Absolute risk reduction

The numerical difference between the risk of an occurrence in the control and treatment groups.

$$(\text{Incidence in treatment group}) - (\text{Incidence in control group})$$

Relative risk reduction

The ratio of the absolute risk reduction to the control group incidence (%):

$$\frac{(\text{Absolute risk reduction})}{(\text{Control incidence})}$$

Relative risk

The ratio of the risk of an occurrence in the treatment group to that in the control group:

$$\frac{(\text{Incidence in treatment group})}{(\text{Incidence in control group})}$$

If the control incidence is low, this can lead to an overestimation of the treatment effect.

Odds ratio

Ratio of the odds of outcome in the treatment group to the odds of outcome in the control group.

Unpaired test

Different patients are studied in each of the intervention groups.

Paired test

The same patient is studied for each intervention, thereby acting as their own control. Matched patients can also be used.

Student's *t*-test

A parametric test for comparison of sample means where

$$t = \frac{\text{Difference between sample means}}{\text{Estimated SE of the difference}}$$

Once a value for t is obtained, it is read from a table to see if it represents a statistically significant difference at the level of probability required, for example $p < 0.05$.

One-tailed test

A statistical test in which the values that will allow rejection of the null hypothesis are located only at one end of the distribution curve.

For example, if a study were to investigate the potential of a new antihypertensive drug, a one-tailed test may be used to look for a decrease but not an increase in BP.

Two-tailed test

A statistical test in which the values that will allow rejection of the null hypothesis are located at either end of the distribution curve.

A study investigating the effect of a drug on serum Na^+ levels could use a two-tailed test to identify both an increase and a decrease. In general, unless you are sure that a variable can only move in one direction, it is wise to use a two-tailed test.

Chi-square (χ^2) test

Compares the frequency of observed results against the frequency that would be expected if there were no difference between the groups.

$$\chi^2 = \Sigma \frac{(O - E)^2}{E}$$

where χ^2 is the chi-square statistic, E is the number of expected occurrences and O is the number of observed occurrences.

It is best demonstrated by constructing a simple 3 × 3 table. You may be provided with a pre-printed table in the examination but be prepared to draw your own.

		Smokers		
		Yes	No	Total
Sex	M	30	60	90
	F	70	20	90
	Total	100	80	180

The numbers in the unshaded portion of the table give you the observed frequency. The expected percentage of smokers if there were no difference between the sexes would be 100/180 (55.6%) smokers and 80/180 (44.4%) non-smokers in each group. To find the actual frequency in each group, this percentage is multiplied by the respective row total.

$$E = \frac{\text{Column total}}{\text{Grand total}} \times \text{Row total}$$

		Smokers Yes	No	Total
Sex	M	30 (50)	60 (40)	90
	F	70 (50)	20 (40)	90
Total		100	80	180

The table now has an expected frequency in parentheses in each cell along with the observed frequency. The calculation $(O - E)^2/E$ is performed for each cell and the results summed to give the χ^2 statistic.

Degrees of freedom for χ^2

Degrees of freedom for a table are calculated in a similar way to those for distributions.

DF = (No. of rows − 1) × (No. of columns − 1)

Therefore for a 2 × 2 table

DF = (2 − 1) × (2 − 1)
DF = 1 × 1
DF = 1

When the χ^2 statistic has been calculated, it is cross-referenced to a table of values together with various degrees of freedom. The table will enable the statistician to see if the groups are statistically different or not.

Fisher's exact test

This is a variation of the χ^2 test that is used when the value for E in any cell is 5 or less.

Correlation

A representation of the degree of association between two variables.

Importantly, this does not identify a cause and effect relationship but simply an association.

Correlation coefficient

A numerical description of how closely the points adhere to the best fit straight line on a correlation plot (*r*).

The value of r lies between ± 1. A value of $+1$ indicates a perfect positive correlation and a value of -1 a perfect negative correlation. A value of 0 indicates that there is no correlation between the two variables.

Regression coefficient

A numerical description of the gradient of the line of best fit using linear regression analysis (*b*).

The regression coefficient allows prediction of one value from another. However, it is only useful when the intercept on the y axis is also known, thereby describing the relationship by fixing the position of the line as for the equation $y = bx + a$.

Positive correlation

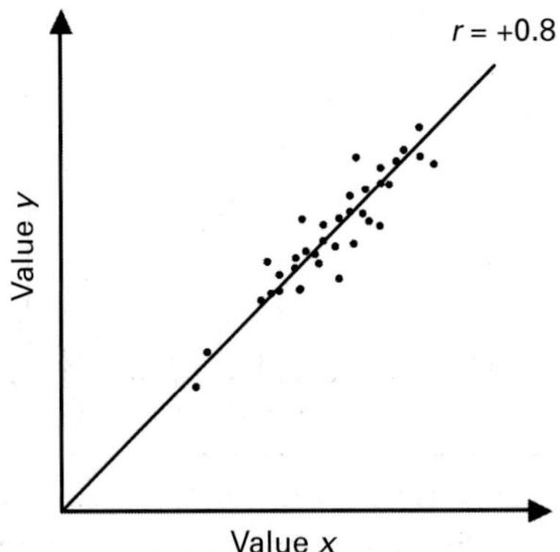

Draw and label the axes. The x axis is traditionally where the independent variable is plotted. Draw a line of best fit surrounded by data points. As the line of best fit has a positive slope, both b and r will be positive. However, r will not be $+1$ as the data points do not lie exactly on the line. In this case r is approximately $+0.8$.

Negative correlation

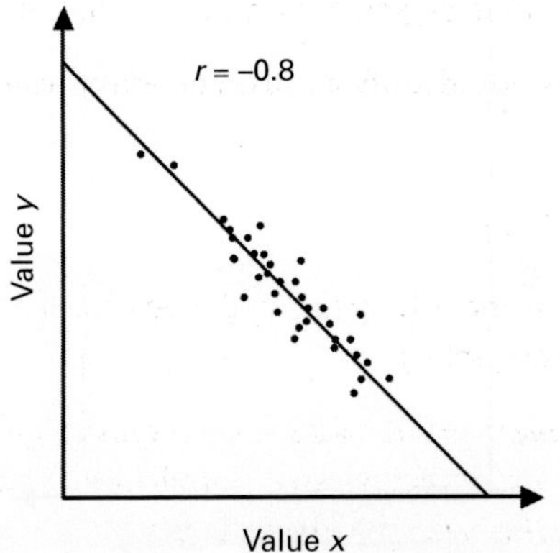

This plot is drawn in exactly the same way but now with a negative slope to the line of best fit. Both b and r will now be negative but, again, r will not be -1 as the data points do not lie exactly on the line. In this case r is approximately -0.8.

Exact negative correlation

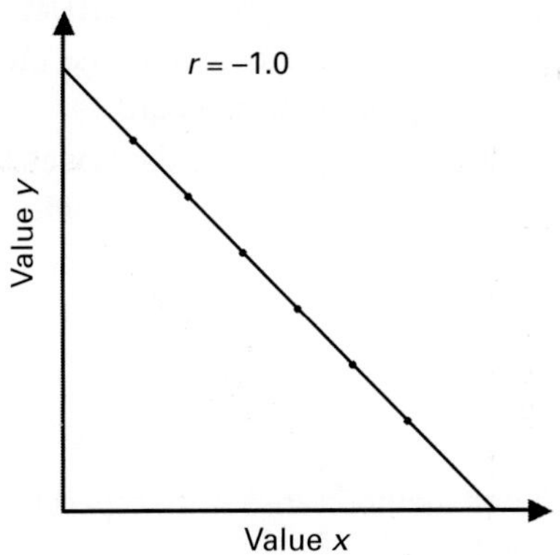

This plot is drawn in the same way as the negative plot but now the line of best fit becomes a line of exact fit. Both b and r will now be negative and r will be -1 as the data points lie exactly on the line.

No correlation

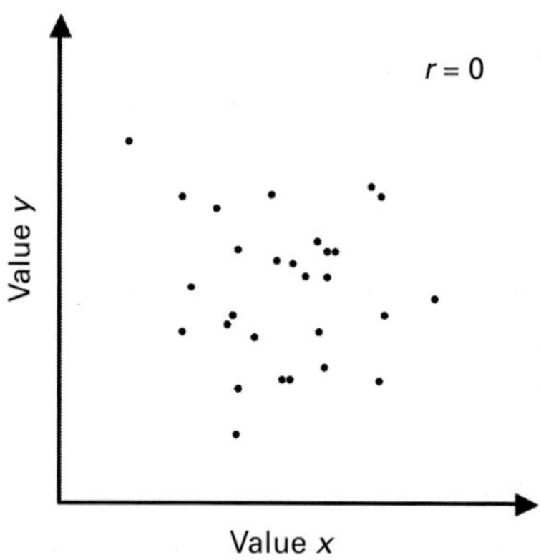

Draw and label the axes as before but note that on this plot there is no meaningful line of best fit as the data points are truly random. It is not possible to give a value for *b* as a line of best fit cannot be generated but the value of *r* is 0.

Bland–Altman plot

The Bland–Altman plot is superior to regression/correlation analysis when used to compare two methods of measurement. It is the method of choice when comparing one method to an agreed gold standard.

The true value being measured by the two methods is assumed to be the average of their readings. This is then plotted against the difference between the two readings at that point. The level of agreement or disagreement at every value is, therefore, obtained and a mean and SD can be calculated.

Bias

The extent to which one method varies with respect to another when the two methods are compared.

The mean difference between methods should ideally be zero. However, if it is felt that the clinical difference between the methods is not significant, then the mean difference can simply be added to or subtracted from the results of one method in order to bring them into line with the gold standard. The amount by which the mean differs from zero is called the bias.

No agreement

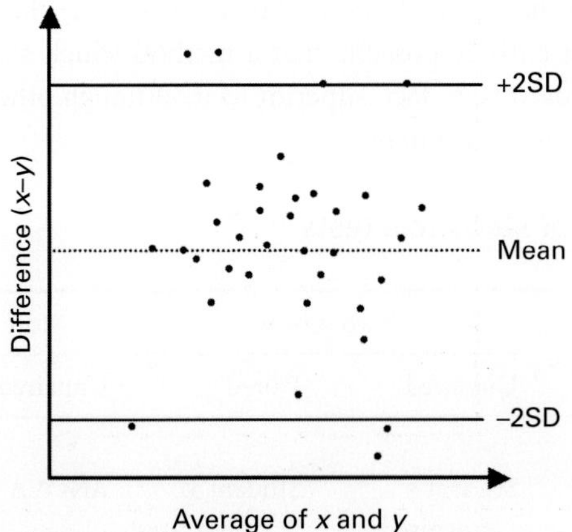

Draw and label the axes as shown. Widely scattered data points as shown suggest no firm comparison between methods *x* and *y*. Demonstrate that ±2SD (95% CI) is wide and the distribution of the points appears arbitrary. Bias can be demonstrated by showing a mean point that does not lie at zero on the *y* axis.

Good agreement

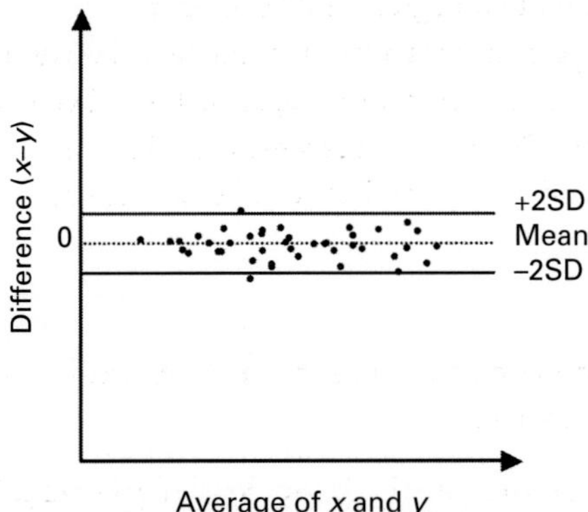

On the same axes draw a tightly packed group of data points centred around a mean difference of zero. The ±2SD should show a narrow range. This plot demonstrates good agreement between the methods used.

Interpretation

The test does not indicate which method is superior, only the level of agreement between them. It is entirely possible that a method which shows no agreement with a current standard is, in fact, superior to it, although other tests would have to be used to determine its suitability.

Reference table of statistical tests

Type of data	Two groups		More than two groups	
	Unpaired	Paired	Unpaired	Paired
Parametric				
Continuous	Student's unpaired *t*-test	Student's paired *t*-test	ANOVA	Paired ANOVA
Non-parametric				
Nominal	χ^2 with Yates' correction	McNemar's test	χ^2	–
Ordinal or numerical	Mann–Whitney *U* test	Wilcoxon signed rank test	Kruskal–Wallis	Friedman

Error and outcome prediction

In medicine, we often try to predict an outcome based on the result of a test. There are various terms used to describe how useful a test is, which may be best understood by reference to a table such as the one below.

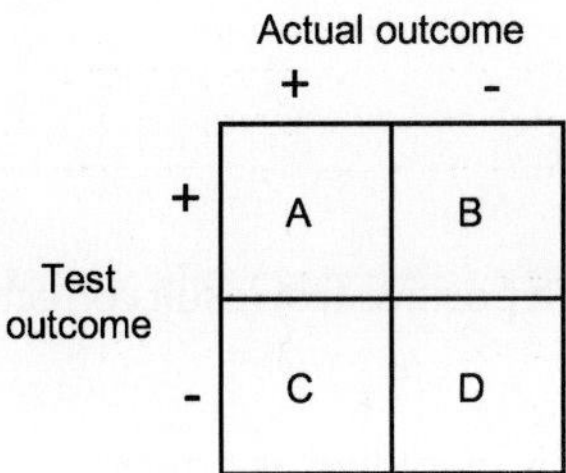

Type I error

The occurrence of a positive test result when the actual value is negative (%).

This type of error equates to box B and is variously described as a type I error, a false-positive error or the α error. A type I error in a study result would lead to the incorrect rejection of the null hypothesis.

Type II error

The occurrence of a negative test result when the actual value is positive (%).

This type of error equates to box C and is variously described as a type II error, a false-negative error or the β error. A type II error in a study result would lead to the incorrect acceptance of the null hypothesis.

Sensitivity

The ability of a test to correctly identify a positive outcome where one exists (%):

$$\frac{\text{The number correctly identified as positive}}{\text{Total number that are actually positive}}$$

or, in the Figure:

$$A/(A+C)$$

Specificity

The ability of a test to correctly identify a negative outcome where one exists (%):

$$\frac{\text{The number correctly identified as negative}}{\text{Total number that are actually negative}}$$

or

$$D/(B + D)$$

Positive predictive value

The certainty with which a positive test result correctly predicts a positive value (%):

$$\frac{\text{The number correctly identified as positive}}{\text{Total number with positive outcome}}$$

or

$$A/(A + B)$$

Negative predictive value

The certainty with which a negative test result correctly predicts a negative value (%):

$$\frac{\text{The number correctly identified as negative}}{\text{Total number with negative outcome}}$$

or

$$D/(C + D)$$

Clinical trials

Phases of clinical trials

Clinical trials will be preceded by in-vitro and animal studies before progressing through the stages shown in the table.

Phase	Description	Numbers
1	Healthy volunteers: pharmacokinetic and pharmacodynamic effects	20–50
2	More pharmacokinetic and dynamic information: different drug doses and frequencies	50–300
3	Randomized controlled trials: comparison with current treatments; assessment of frequent side effects	250–1000 +
PRODUCT LICENCE		
4	Postmarketing surveillance: rare side effects	2000–10 000 +

Trial design flow sheet

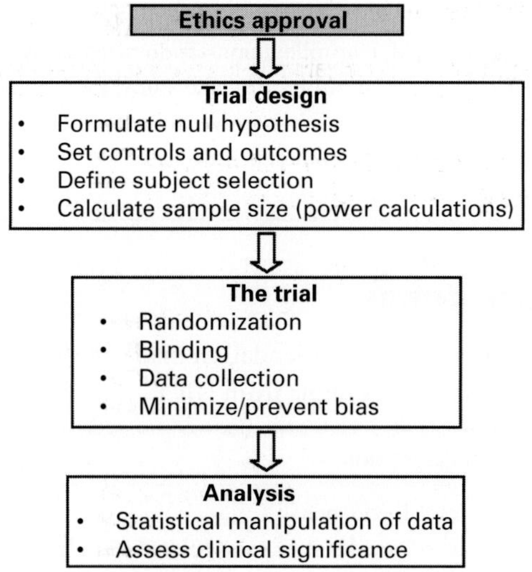

Evidence-based medicine

Evidence-based medicine

The use of current best evidence, clinical expertise and patient values to make decisions about the care of individual patients.

Levels of evidence

In this era of evidence-based medicine, there needs to be a method of categorizing the available evidence to indicate how useful it is. The following system is the one used by the UK National Institute for Health and Clinical Excellence (NICE). Other organizations that produce guidelines may use slightly different systems but the hierarchy of usefulness remains the same. The levels of evidence are based on study design, with some systems, such as this one, subdividing the grades further depending on the methodological quality of individual studies.

Level	Evidence description
1a	Systematic review or meta-analysis of one or more randomized controlled trials (RCT)
1b	At least one RCT
2a	At least one well-designed, controlled, non-randomized study
2b	At least one well-designed quasi-experimental study; for example a cohort study
3	Well-designed non-experimental descriptive studies; for example comparative, correlation or case–control studies, or case series
4	Expert opinion

Grade of recommendations

Similarly, the strength of any recommendation made on the basis of the evidence can be categorized. This is an example from NICE.

Grade	Recommendation description
A	Based directly on level 1 evidence
B	Based directly on level 2 evidence or extrapolated from level 1 evidence
C	Based directly on level 3 evidence or extrapolated from level 1 or level 2 evidence
D	Based directly on level 4 evidence or extrapolated from level 1, level 2 or level 3 evidence
GPP	Good practice point based on the view of the Guideline Development Group

An alternative is to think in terms of 'do it' or 'don't do it', based on conclusions drawn from high-quality evidence or 'probably do it' or 'probably don't do it' based on moderate quality evidence. Low-quality evidence leads to uncertainly and inability to make a recommendation.

Meta-analysis

> **A statistical technique that combines the results of several independent studies that address a similar research hypothesis.**

Meta-analysis aims to increase the statistical power of the available evidence by combining the results of smaller trials together using specific statistical methods. The validity of the meta-analysis will depend on the quality of the evidence on which it is based and how homogeneous or comparable the samples are. Combining very heterogeneous study populations can lead to bias.

Forest plot

> **A graphical representation of the results of a meta-analysis.**

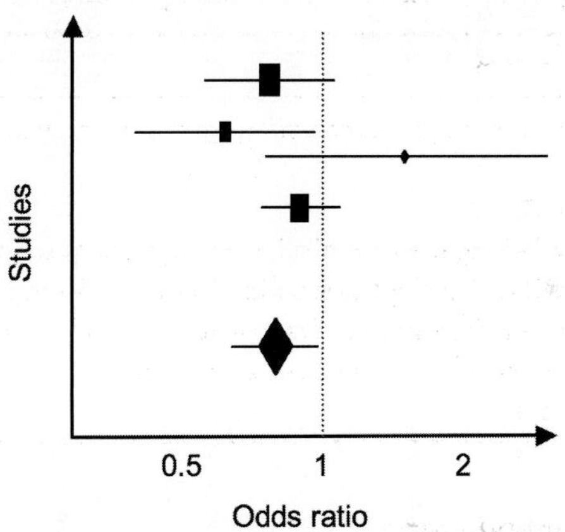

Begin by drawing and labelling the axes as shown. Draw a vertical line from 1 on the x axis. This is the line of no effect. The results of the individual trials are shown as boxes with the size of the box relating to the size of the trial and its position relating to the result of the trial. The lines are usually the 95% confidence intervals. The combined result is shown at the bottom of all the trials as a diamond, the size of which represents the combined numbers from all the trials. The result can be considered statistically significant if the confidence intervals of the combined result do not cross the line of no effect.

Appendix

Intravenous induction agents

	Thiopental	Methohexital	Propofol	Ketamine	Etomidate
Chemical composition	Thiobarbiturate	Oxybarbiturate	2,6 Diisopropylphenol	Phenylcyclidine derivative	Imidazole ester
Dose (mg.kg^{-1})	3–7	1–1.5	1–2	1–2 i.v., 5–10 i.m.	0.3
p*K*a	7.6	7.9	11.0	7.5	4.0
pH in solution	10.5	11	6–8.5	3.5–5.5	8.1
Volume of distribution (l.kg^{-1})	2.5	2.0	4.0	3.0	3.0
Protein binding (%)	80	60	98	25	75
Racemic	✓	✓	x	✓	✓
Action	↑duration of $GABA_A$ opening, leading to ↑ Cl^- current		Stimulates GABA; inhibits NMDA	Inhibits NMDA and opioid μ receptors (stimulates κ and δ)	Stimulates GABA
Metabolism	Oxidation		Glucuronidation Hydroxylation	*N*-Demethylation Hydroxylation	Plasma and hepatic esterases
Metabolites	Active	Minimal activity	Inactive	Active	Inactive
Clearance (ml.kg^{-1}.min^{-1})	3.5	11	30–60	17	10–20
Elimination rate (t_{elim}) (h)	6–15	3–5	5–12	2	1–4
Hypersensitivity	Anaphylaxis 1:20 000	More common than thiopental but less severe		Rashes in 15%	Rare

Intravenous induction agents: physiological effects

	Thiopental	Methohexital	Propofol	Ketamine	Etomidate
Blood pressure	↓	↓	↓↓	↑	↔
Cardiac output	↓	↓	↓↓	↑	↔
Heart rate	↑	↑	↓→	↑	↔
Systemic vascular resistance	↕	↕	↓↓	↔	↔
Respiratory rate	↓	↓	↓	↑	↓
Intracranial pressure	↓	↓	↓	↑	↔
Intraocular pressure	↓	↓	↓	↑	↔
Pain on injection	No	Yes	Yes	No	Yes
Nausea/vomiting	No	No	No	Yes	Yes
Miscellaneous	Intra-arterial injection → crystallization	↓ Fit threshold	? Toxic in children (metabolic acidosis and bradycardia)	↑ Salivation; 'dissociative anaesthesia'	Adrenal suppression

Inhalational anaesthetic agents

	Halothane	Isoflurane	Enflurane	Sevoflurane	Desflurane	Nitrous oxide
Relative molecular mass (kDa)	197	184.5	184.5	200.1	168	44
Boiling point (°C)	50.2	48.5	56.5	58.5	23.5	−88
Saturated vapour pressure at 20 °C (kPa)	32.3	33.2	23.3	22.7	89.2	5200
Blood:gas	2.4	1.4	1.8	0.7	0.45	0.47
Oil:gas	224	98	98	80	29	1.4
Minimum alveolar concentration	0.75	1.17	1.68	1.8–2.2	6.6	105
Odour	Non-irritant	Irritant	Non-irritant	Non-irritant	Pungent	Odourless
Metabolized (%)	20	0.2	2	3.5	0.02	0.01
Metabolites	Trifluoroacetic acid, Cl^-, Br^-	Trifluoroacetic acid, F^-,	Inorganic and organic fluorides	Inorganic and organic fluorides; compounds A–E	Trifluoroacetic acid	Nitrogen

Xenon: 131 kDa; boiling point −108 °C; blood:gas solubility coefficient 14; oil:gas solubility coefficient 1.9; MAC 71; odourless.

Inhalational agents: physiological effects

	Halothane	Isoflurane	Enflurane	Sevoflurane	Desflurane	Nitrous oxide
Contractility	↓↓↓	↓	↓↓	↓	↔	↓
Heart rate	↓↓	↑↑	↑	↔	↑ (↑↑ > 1.5 MAC)	↔
Systemic vascular resistance	↓	↓↓	↓	↓	↓↓	
Blood pressure	↓↓	↓↓	↓↓	↓	↓↓	–
Sensitivity to catecholamines	↑↑↑	–	↑	–	–	
Respiratory rate	↑	↑↑	↑↑	↑↑	↑↑	↑
Tidal volume	↓	↓↓	↓↓↓	↓	↓↓	↓
$P\text{aCO}_2$	↔	↑↑	↑↑↑	↑	↑↑	↔
Bronchodilatation	Yes		Yes	Yes	Irritant	–
Cerebral blood flow	↑↑↑	↑ (Yes MAC > 1)	↑	Preserves autoregulation	↑	↑
Cerebral metabolic O_2 rate	↓	↓	↓	↓	↓	↓
Electroencephalography	Burst suppression	Burst suppression	Epileptiform activity	Burst suppression	Burst suppression	
Uterus	Some relaxation	Some relaxation	Some relaxation	Some relaxation	Some relaxation	
Muscle relaxation	Some	Significant	Significant	Significant	Significant	
Analgesia	Some	Some	Some	Some	Some	
Miscellaneous	Hepatotoxicity; stored in 0.01% thymol; light sensitive	Coronary steal?; maintains renal blood flow	Hepatotoxic; avoid in renal impairment	Renal toxicity		Oxidizes cobalt ion in vitamin B_{12}

MAC, minimum alveolar concentration.

Opioids[a]

	Morphine	Diamorphine	Codeine	Pethidine	Fentanyl	Alfentanil	Remifentanil
Chemical composition		Diacetylmorphine	Methylmorphine	← Synthetic phenylpiperidines →			
p*K*a	8.0	7.6	8.2	8.7	8.4	6.5	7.1
Relative lipid solubility	1	250		30	600	90	20
Relative potency	1	2	0.1	0.1	100	10–20	100
Protein binding (%)	35	40	7	60	83	90	70
Volume of distribution ($l.kg^{-1}$)	3.5	5	5.4	4.0	4.0	0.6	0.3
Oral bioavailability (%)	25–30	Low	50 (20–80)	50	33	N/A	N/A
Metabolism	Glucuronidation; *N*-demethylation	Ester hydrolysis to morphine	Glucuronidation; demethylation (CYP2D6)	Ester hydrolysis; *N*-demethylation	*N*-Dealkylation, then hydroxylation	*N*-Demethylation	Plasma and tissue esterases
Clearance ($ml.kg^{-1}.min^{-1}$)	16	3.1	23	12	13	6	40
Elimination rate (min)	170	5 ($t_{1/2}$)	170	210	190	100	10

[a] Opioids are bases.

Local anaesthetics[a]

	Esters (-COO-)		Amides (-NHCO-)				
	Procaine	Amethocaine	Lidocaine	Prilocaine	Bupivicaine	Ropivicaine	Mepivicaine
Relative potency[b]	1	8	2	2	8	8	2
Onset[c]	Slow	Slow	Fast	Fast	Medium	Medium	Slow
Duration[d]	Short	Long	Medium	Medium	Long	Long	Medium
Maximum dose ($mg.kg^{-1}$)	12	1.5	3	6	2	3.5	5
Toxic plasma level ($\mu g.ml^{-1}$)			>5	>5	>1.5	>4	>5
p*K*a	8.9	8.5	7.9	7.7	8.1	8.1	7.6
Protein bound (%)	6	75	70	55	95	94	77
Relative lipid solubility	1	200	150	50	1000	300	50
Volume of distribution (l)			92	191	73	59	
Metabolism	By esterases to *para*-aminobenzoic acid (allergenic)		← By hepatic amidases →				
Clearance ($l.min^{-1}$)			1	2.4	.6	0.82	
Elimination rate (min)			100	100	160	120	115

[a] Local anaesthetics are weak bases. They have hydrophilic plus hydrophobic components linked by an ester or amide group (hence classification). Local anaesthetics can act as vasodilators; prilocaine > lignocaine > bupivicaine > ropivicaine.
[b] Potency is related to lipid solubility.
[c] Speed of onset is related to pKa.
[d] Duration of action is related to protein binding.

Non-depolarizing muscle relaxants

	Aminosteroids			Benzylisoquinoliniums				
	Vecuronium	Rocuronium	Pancuronium	Atracurium	Cis-atracurium	Mivacurium	Gallamine	Tubocurare
Structure	Monoquaternary	Monoquaternary	Bisquaternary	10 stereoisomers		3 stereoisomers		Monoquaternary
Dose (mg.kg^{-1})	0.1	0.6	0.1	0.5	0.2	0.2	2.0	0.5
Onset	Medium	Rapid	Medium	Medium	Medium	Medium	Rapid	Slow
Duration	Medium	Medium	Long	Medium	Medium	Short	Medium	Long
Cardiovascular effects	↓ HR	–	↑ HR	–	–	–	↑ HR	↓ BP
Histamine release	–	–	–	Mild	Rare	Mild	Rare	Common
Protein bound (%)	10	10	20–60	15	15	10	10	30–50
Volume of distribution (l.kg^{-1})	0.2	0.2	0.3	0.15	0.15	0.2–0.3	0.2	0.3
Metabolism (%)	20[a]	< 5[a]	30[a]	90[b]	95	90	0	0
Elimination in bile (%)	70	60	20	0	0	0	0	30
Elimination in urine (%)	30	40	80	10	5	5	100	70
Renal failure	←——Prolonged action——→			–	–	–	←Prolonged action→	

HR, heart rate; BP, blood pressure.

[a] By deacetylation.

[b] By Hoffman degradation and ester hydrolysis.

Intravenous fluids: crystalloids

	Na^+ (mmol.l^{-1})	K^+ (mmol.l^{-1})	Ca^{2+} (mmol.l^{-1})	Cl^- (mmol.l^{-1})	HCO_3^- (mmol.l^{-1})	Osm (mmol.l^{-1})	pH	Glucose (g.l^{-1})
0.9% Saline	154	0	0	154	0	300	5	0
5% Dextrose	0	0	0	0	0	280	4	50
10% Dextrose	0	0	0	0	0	560	4	100
4% Dextrose, 0.18% saline	31	0	0	31	0	255	4.5	40
Hartmann's solution	131	5	2	111	29	278	6	0
8.4% $NaHCO_3$	1000	0	0	0	1000	2000	8	0

Intravenous fluids: colloids

	Composition	M_W (kDa)	Na^+ (mmol.l^{-1})	K^+ (mmol.l^{-1})	Ca^{2+} (mmol.l^{-1})	Mg^{2+} (mmol.l^{-1})	Cl^- (mmol.l^{-1})	Osm (mmol.l^{-1})	pH
Gelofusine	Succinylated gelatin	30–35	154	0.4	0.4	0.4	125	279	7.4
Haemaccel	Polygelines	30–35	145	5.1	6.25	0	145	301	7.3
Hydroxyethyl starch (HES)	Esterified amylopectin	450	154	0	0	0	154		
Dextran 70	Polysaccharides in 5% dextrose	70	0	0	0	0	0	287	3.5–7
HES 4.5%	Fractionation of plasma	69	100–160	<2	0	0	100–160	270–300	6.4–7.4
HES 20%		69	50–120	<10	0	0	<40	135–138	6.4–7.4

M_W, relative molecular mass.

Vaughan–Williams classification of antiarrhythmic drugs

Class	Action	Effect on cardiac conduction	Examples
I	Sodium channel blockade		
Ia		Prolongs refractory period	Quinidine, procainamide, disopyramide
Ib		Shortens refractory period	Lidocaine, mexilitine, phenytoin
Ic		None	Flecainide, propafenone
II	Beta blockade	Slows atrioventricular conduction	Propranolol, atenolol, esmolol
III	Potassium channel blockade	Slows atrioventricular conduction	Amiodarone, sotolol
IV	Calcium channel blockade	Prolongs refractory period	Verapamil, diltiazem

Gases: physical properties

Gas	M_w (kDa)	BP (°C)	CT (°C)	CP (bar)	η	ρ
Nitrogen	28	−196	−147	34	17.6	1.165
Oxygen	32	−182	−118	50	20.4	1.331
Carbon dioxide	44	−78.5	31	74	14.7	1.831
Air	29	−195	−149	38	18.2	1.196
Nitrous oxide	44	−88	36.5	72	14.6	1.83
Helium	4	−269	−268	2.3	19.6	0.166

M_W, relative molecular mass; BP, boiling point; CT, critical temperature; CP, critical pressure; η, viscosity; ρ, density.

Body fluid composition

Component[a]	Plasma	Interstitial	Intracellular
Percentage total body water[b]	5	15	40
Na^+ ($mmol.l^{-1}$)	145	140	10
K^+ ($mmol.l^{-1}$)	4	5	155
Ca^{2+} ($mmol.l^{-1}$)	3	2	<1
Mg^{2+} ($mmol.l^{-1}$)	1	2	40
Cl^- ($mmol.l^{-1}$)	110	112	3
HCO_3^- ($mmol.l^{-1}$)	26	28	7
Others[c] ($mmol.l^{-1}$)	7	9	150
Proteins ($mmol.l^{-1}$)	10	–	45

[a] The numbers will vary depending on the source but the cations (positively charged ions) should always equal the anions (negatively charged ions).
[b] Water is 60% of total body weight in an adult male.
[c] Include sulphates, phosphates and inorganic acids.

Daily nutritional requirements for a 70 kg male

	Requirement per kg body weight
Energy	
Calories (kcal)	30–40
Food components(g)	
Glucose	3–4
Fat	1
Protein	1
Nitrogen	0.2
Fluid (ml)	30–40
Electrolytes (mmol)	
Sodium	1–2
Potassium	1
Calcium	18
Magnesium	12
Chloride	1
Phosphate	18

Urinary electrolytes in renal failure: this table is always difficult to recall but try to remember that in intrinsic renal failure the kidney is unable to concentrate urine effectively and so a poor quality, dilute urine is produced

	Pre-renal	Renal
Urine ($mmol.l^{-1}$)		
Osmolarity	>450 (concentrated)	<350 (dilute, poor quality)
Sodium	<15 (Na^+ retention)	>40 (Na^+ loss)
Urea	>250 (excreting lots)	<160 (not excreting much)
Urine: plasma concentrations[a]		
Osmolarity	>2 (urine more concentrated)	<1.5 (urine less concentrated)
Creatinine	>40	<40
Urea	>8	<3

[a] If the ratio is high, it means that there is relatively more of the substance in the urine.

Types of muscle fibre

Fibre	Slow oxidative (type I)	Fast oxidative (type IIa)	Fast glycolytic (type IIb)
Diameter	Small	Intermediate	Large
Conduction velocity	Slow	Fast	Fast
Twitch	Long	Short	Short
Colour	Red	Red	White
Myoglobin	+++	+++	+
Source of ATP	Oxidative phosphorylation	Oxidative phosphorylation	Glycolysis
Glycogen and glycolytic enzymes	+	++	+++
Fatiguability	+	++	+++

Index